ALLICIN

The Heart of Garlic

A fungal nail infection similar to that which affects tens of millions of Americans before treatment

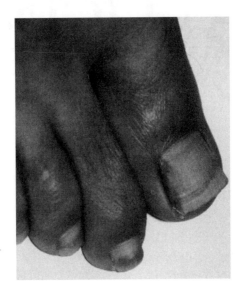

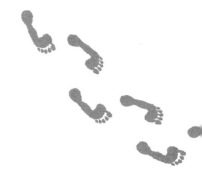

ALLICIN

The Heart of Garlic

Nature's aid to healing the human body

By Peter Josling

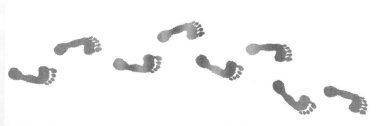

ALLICIN
The heart of garlic

Nature's aid to healing the human body

How to use allicin for superior health benefits

Peter Josling
Director of The Garlic Centre

NWI Publishing   Callahan, Florida

Copyright NWI Publishing 2004

Printed in the United States of America
First Edition

ISBN 1-900052-10-5

Disclaimer: This book is not intended as a substitute for medical diagnosis or treatment.
Anyone who has an existing disease should consult a physician before initiating any change
in treatment or before beginning a new course of treatment.
For ordering information please call 1-877-763-7779

SPECIAL INFORMATION

All the remedies discussed in this book relate ONLY to allicin containing products that have been
manufactured and supplied by AXI Limited. The extract referred to as a powder capsule,
a liquid or a creme must contain Allisure® as the primary active ingredient.
If this is not stated, then the product will not contain allicin and may not perform as you hope.
Please refer to the web site www.allisure.com for further details.

Table of Contents

Introduction	The microbe hits back!	7
Chapter One	A brief history lesson	15
Chapter Two	A brief chemistry lesson	19
Chapter Three	A-Z of medical uses	31
Chapter Four	How does allicin work and what else can it do?	142
Chapter Five	Allicin and cancer prevention	145
Chapter Six	Conclusion	150
Bibliography		153
Appendix	Fungal species killed by allicin Bacterial species killed by allicin Viral species killed by allicin Parasites killed by allicin Other diseases where allicin may be helpful	155
Index		160

INTRODUCTION

The microbe hits back!

The well-worn phrase, "Garlic is good for you," is acknowledged the world over, and perhaps many more people in the last few years have begun to realize that this is most certainly a truism. I can't think of any other plant that has such an established and magnificent track record for performing good deeds. Dating back to the early Egyptians and Sumerians over 5,000 years ago, this remarkable herb was quickly established as the most adaptable and proficient food widely used for both its culinary and medicinal benefits.

Garlic is used by every culture the world over, referenced in the Holy Bible (*Numbers 10:23*) and yet still, in the 21st century, reveals its true potential to conquer modern-day problems. Garlic contains many beneficial components, and over the last 10 to 15 years an enormous amount of research has been published on the properties of various breakdown components that are formed when fresh garlic is cut, crushed, chopped or processed.

Of these well-known and categorized sulfur-containing chemicals, it is **allicin** that stands out head and shoulders above the rest, showing the most exciting, interesting and beneficial properties. Now with the advent of new technology, for the first time ever it is possible to produce stabilized allicin on a commercial scale. This has led to research confirming the most incredible spectrum of activity against today's most pressing problems— resistant bacteria, viral and fungal infections, and microorganisms that have long been the scourge of modern man.

We never expect to become infected by these clever killers and yet every surface we touch, every person we meet, every animal we pet, everywhere we go, we are ambushed by microbes. General Custer had a chance, but the way we are going we will ALL eventually succumb to infection! We thought we had "conquered" killers like tuberculosis, smallpox, typhus, pertussis, dysentery, hepatitis, shigella, amebic dysentery and many other infectious diseases with the advent of modern-day antibiotic therapy. Leading physicians prematurely declared that the war against microbes was won, yet they have returned with a vengeance. London, England is now the TB capital of Europe. New York City has re-opened special hospitals to quarantine infectious patients, and it is estimated that in Russia there are over 4 million people with multi-drug resistant diseases who are walking around the streets of Moscow and St. Petersburg happily spreading the pool of infection.

Infectious diseases are quickly returning to their former prominence, and we are unable to stop them with chemical pharmaceutical agents.

It is estimated that the number of bacteria, viral and fungal pathogens to be found either in or around every human being is infinite. This is why, after 70 years of producing pharmaceutical antibiotics, recent surveys indicate that 90% of visits to doctor's offices are infection related. Over 1 million metric tons of antibiotics have been dispersed into the bioshpere in the past 50 years to cure these infections, half for human use and half for animal use, which means that the indigenous bacteria of **all** living species are richly populated with resistant bacteria that we cannot get rid of. Is it any wonder that public health physicians are worried?

Why are we losing the battle?

Recent news reports show that bacteria may send messages to each other about resisting antibiotic poisoning (*Medicine Today, June 2002*). In fact, bacterial signalling is going on all the time, all over your body, especially in your mouth and guts. Finding ways of interfering with this signalling process are the latest developments in the antibiotic arms race.

Major consequences of these bacterial conversations are biological buildings! Among the more extraordinary sights visible through the new $350,000 confocal laser scanning microscopes, which allow objects to be viewed almost in 3D, are what have been dubbed "Slime Cities"— armoured defensive communities where bacteria live and reproduce, safe from antibiotics, your immune system and other predators.

Known technically as biofilms, thesse are currently the target of intense research since it has become increasingly clear that biofilms lie at the root of some of our most intractable conditions. The American Centres for Disease Control and Prevention estimate that 65% of human bacterial infections involve biofilms. Not only are they responsible for tooth decay and gum disease, but they also cause many of the problems associated with cystic fibrosis, ear infections and infections of the prostate gland and heart. They cause an estimated expenditure of $6 billion a year in the USA by causing hard-to-treat infections on catheters, artificial heart valves and other medical implants. Similarly, irrational prescribing causes an over usage of the very agents used to remove these infectious organisms. It is estimated that every year in the United States ten million adults seek treatment for acute bronchitis. Most are given antibiotics, even though the pathogens involved in most cases are viruses, so antibiotics won't work.

We tend to think of bacteria as primitive single-celled creatures, but when organized into a biofilm they differentiate, communicate, cooperate and deploy collective defences against antibiotics. In short, they behave like a multicellular organism.

In fact, bacteria from biofilms were among the first ever to be seen through a microscope when pioneer Anton Leeuwenhoek looked at the plaque—a biofilm—scraped from his own teeth in the late 1600s. But it wasn't until the 1970s that scientists began to appreciate just how complex these micro-slime cities are. Plaque, for instance, is founded on a base of dense opaque slime about 5 micrometres thick. Above this vast colonies of bacteria, shaped like mushrooms or cones, rise to a thickness between 100 to 200 micrometres.

Enclosed within their highly effective, defensive wall of slime live communities of many bacterial strains. One researcher described them as: "'Cities' are permeated at all levels by a network of channels through which water, bacterial garbage, nutrients, enzymes, metabolites and oxygen travel to and fro."

"The bacteria inside a biofilm or slime city, which are 15% bacterial cells and 85% slime, are 1000 times less likely to succumb to antibiotics than bacteria in free floating state."

The notion that bacteria can talk to each other was first proposed over 30 years ago by scientists studying "glow in the dark" bacteria, such as *Vibro fischeri*, that live in the specialised "light organs" of certain squid and marine fish. Bacteria do not glow as individuals swimming freely, but when enough of them come together as a group, their illuminations are visible. It seems this must be how they let each other know when enough of them have been gathered. It wasn't until the 1980s that researchers identified the chemical they each put out—AHL (acyl-homoserine lactone). The more bacteria there are in one place, the higher the level of AHL. A level of AHL above a certain threshold will trigger the luminescence, this is usually referred to as Quorum Sensing.

Gradually a better understanding of just how biofilms fight off antibiotics is emerging. The bacteria benefit from pooling their effects. For instance, in a biofilm some bacteria can produce an enzyme that inactivates the antiseptic, hydrogen peroxide, but a single bacterium can't make enough to save itself. Another factor is that even if an antibiotic does get through and kill off some bacterial inhabitants, a substantial number are likely to survive. This is because bacteria exist in a spectrum of physiological states ranging from rapidly-growing to dormant. Antibiotics usually target some activity like cell division. This means that the dormant bacteria will usually live to fight another day.

Dr. Richard Novick has found that *Staphylococcus aureus* can be divided into four different types, each with slightly different signalling molecules. The molecules used by one type stimulated activity in its own group, but inhibited it in the others. This is an example of the way bacteria compete with each other. This particular bacterium is a worry to virtually every health-care establishment in the Western World, as it has developed a number of strains that are resistant to ALL pharmaceutical antibiotics, even vancomycin, a toxic parenteral drug that is usually reserved as a last resort (see MRSA in the medical section Chapter 3).

❝It has been estimated that 40% of proteins in bacterial walls are different in "city dwellers" from those that are "free ranging." This implies that some of the proteins identified in cultures, and targeted by antibiotics, just aren't there in city dwellers.❞

Bacteria are infinitly adaptable and can find ways of slipping under the enemy radar, or in this case, avoiding the immune system. For instance, in *Vibrio cholerae*, the bacterium that causes cholera, the same genes involved in regulating quorum sensing also turn on the toxin production (*Proc Natl Acad Sci, 5 March 2002*). This strategy is valuable because few toxic bacteria might alert the immune system and be rapidly engulfed. By waiting to turn on toxicity until there are enough of them, they have a better chance of overwhelming the host's defences.

Most of the work on quorum sensing has concentrated on chemicals that allow members of the same species to talk to one another. While Dr. Bonnie Bassler at Princeton University was working on the luminous bacteria that led to the finding of quorum sensing in the first place, she made the remarkable discovery that signals from other bacteria could also turn on their lights. It seems that bacteria have some sort of Esperanto—a language for communicating between species (*Nature, 31 January 2002*)—which involves a protein known as A1-2. Exactly what this system is used for isn't clear yet. Among the bacteria that infect humans, those found to produce A1-2 include *Escherichia coli* (food poisoning), *Haemophilus influenzae* (pneumonia and meningitis), *Helicobacter pylori* (peptic ulcers), *Yersinia pestis* (bubonic plague) and *Staphylococcus aureus* (pneumonia, meningitis and toxic shock syndrome). **ALL of these bacteria can be killed by low concentrations of allicin.**

Allicin is mother nature's defender! Allicin can penetrate a biofilm, destroy a wide range of bacterial species, wipe out fungal infections, boost an underactive immune system, reduce cholesterol and blood pressure levels, prevent viral infections, kill off parasites, remove protozoal organisms, vasodilate when necessary, prevent the release of histamine, prevent mosquitoes from attacking—yes, ALL of this from an agent that is produced naturally from fresh garlic!

Research is currently underway, using the latest technology, that allows us to blast apart a bacterial cell and detect exactly which proteins and enzymes it can produce. Then the same species is treated with allicin liquid or powder, blasted apart again and analyzed to see which proteins and enzymes have been disabled, consequently inactive and unable to infect us. We already know that allicin is capable of penetrating bacterial cell walls and preventing the release of many enzymes that are toxic to humans. Chapter 4 and the appendix to this book describe an immense spectrum of activity for allicin powder, liquid and creme formulations, against bacterial species, viral infections, fungal and protozoal disease, as well as a large number of parasital problems.

In this book you will read how allicin, now referred to as "Nature's Antibiotic" can kill TB, smallpox, MRSA, Acinetobacter and many, many more threats to your health. With the additional benefit of strengthening your immune system to prevent further attack while not disrupting or destroying your existing healthy bacteria. Allicin can help your body in many different ways. You will also learn how to prevent the common cold, remove troublesome cold sores, combat athlete's foot and protect yourself from further infection.

As I was writing this book, it became necessary to produce a further updated version, since many studies on allicin powder capsules, liquid, creme, and allicin added to a wide range of other active raw ingredients is underway. Even the US National Institute of Health has recently instructed the NIAID (National Institute for Allergy and Infectious Diseases) and USAMRIID (United States Army Medical Research Institute of Infectious Disease) to secure enough material to test allicin, in all its new formulations, against West Nile virus, Vaccinia, smallpox, cowpox, Rocky Mountain Spotted Fever and Severe Acute Respiratory Syndrome (SARS). Why? Because it will probably work!

Aside from this crucial need for a natural antibiotic/ antifungal/antiviral, allicin therapy has begun to move into the prevention and treatment areas of the world's two biggest killer diseases: cancer and coronary heart disease. These modern-day killers, particularly in the developed world, account for over 50 percent of all deaths recorded in the Western World, with the UK and America particularly high up the scale.

Yet the paradox is that those nations where garlic consumption, both cooked and raw, is a strong part of the culture and daily life show much lower coronary death rates and significant protection from cancer. Obviously, there are many other factors involved, but this book, for the first time, details the results of medically approved studies and confirms what great physicians, herbalists and healers have suggested for thousands of years, namely, something that garlic produces is good for human health. Now, at long last, after 80 years of trying to release the Mother substance—the HEART of garlic-we can finally deliver ALLICIN in sufficient quantity to YOUR body! In writing this book I should like to record my grateful thanks to Dr. Ron Cutler from the University of East London for his many contributions and to Chuck Crismier for helping me with the manuscript.

Do please remember that before following any of the suggested uses for allicin in this book, readers are asked to give consideration to any health problems they may have and should refer to a general practitioner or physician for advice. Many of the remedies recorded, however, do work, so start looking around the globe for 100% allicin-yielding products that are trademarked as containing Allisure® extract.

Kindest regards,

Peter Josling
Director, The Garlic Centre

CHAPTER ONE

A brief history lesson

Garlic has a reputation as a "herb all heal" established over many thousands of years. Of all the numerous herbs, spices and seasonings, it must be not only the best known to most people, but the most useful plant across many walks of life. The history of garlic and its use as a valuable food and restorative medicine dates back to Egyptian times, but was also popular with the Babylonians and Hebrews. The great pyramid at Giza has an inscription showing how much garlic and onion was consumed by the workers who built the pyramids. It is also reported that garlic was the cause of the first-ever industrial strike. When the ruling Egyptians removed the daily ration of garlic given to the workers to ward off disease and build strength, they immediately put down their tools and refused to continue until the rations were restored! Three thousand five hundred years ago this humble bulb was revered. The Egyptians often left clay models of garlic in ordinary graves. When Tutenkhamun's tomb was excavated in 1922 by Howard Carter, he found six bulbs of garlic carefully placed in the tomb—probably to ward off evil spirits.

The Egyptians knew well the power of garlic. According to record, they were renowned for growing vast quantities of grain and therefore made enormous amounts of bread—the staple of an average diet in those days. This often led to problems with tooth decay, since constant milling of the flour led to fine grains of silica breaking down from the sandstone mill-wheels. The only solution was to use the pungent qualities of garlic, ground to a paste, and applied straight to the aching tooth! This rather hot climate was also infested with mosquitoes, gnats and other biting insects, many of which could harbour malaria and other infectious diseases of the time, but once again garlic was able to repel these nasty beasties!

As time passed, the uses of garlic in medicine flourished, and many great physicians and philosophers recalled the usefulness and effectiveness of garlic. Hippocrates, Homer, Aristotle, Pliny, Galen, Virgil and Muhammad all believed garlic to have many useful properties. The Greek and Roman armies were fed garlic to build strength, and the first Olympian athletes consumed vast quantities before a competition to build stamina and keep free from illness. Garlic was thought to be food fit for a god or goddess, and was placed ceremoniously on piles of stones at crossroads for the goddess Hecate.

Since early civilization, garlic has been used by all the leading cultures around the developing world. Nowhere has garlic been more used than in China, in both cooking and medicine. The Chinese call garlic "suan," which is written as a single sign indicating the earliest recognition amongst the Chinese culture. Traditionally, garlic was used as an aid to long life, known both as a "healing" and a "heating" herb, having many benefits to the circulation, for tumours, tuberculosis, coughs, colds, infections and wound healing.

The Romans introduced garlic to Britain in the Dark Ages, where it was grown in monastery gardens. By the Middle Ages, garlic was well established, although not exclusively loved by all. It was around this time that legends began, reporting the magical properties of garlic and its renowned ability to ward off evil spirits and, in particular, vampires! First thought to have been grown in Elizabethan country gardens in 16th century England, garlic became known as peasant's food. The odour was thought to be offensive and not something of which the middle and upper classes should approve of. Here, garlic acquired the country name of Poor Man's Treacle, derived from the Greek word for "antidote," which in Latin was *theiracus*. It was also commonly known as Devil's Posy and Witch Poison, since it was thought to fight off evil. Another name that became synonymous with garlic was Camphor of the Poor due to its strong odour.

Since the World Wars, garlic has been looked upon with increased favour. During the First World War, the British Government offered to pay a shilling a pound to farmers for growing garlic throughout the UK. Garlic's medicinal properties were being used to fight off dysentery and act as an aid towards healing and preventing bacterial infection in the wounded soldiers. During the Second World War, garlic was again used extensively for its antibiotic qualities.

Garlic is a plant whose origins lie in the steppes of Central Asia where it grows wild. As a member of the lily family (*Liliaceae*), its botanical name is *Allium sativum* (for the cultivated variety). Other close members of the family include the onion (*Allium cepa*), chives (*Allium schoenoprasum*), the leek (*Allium porrum*) and the shallot (*Allium ascolonium*). It is also related to the autumn crocus, the bluebell, aloe vera and lily of the valley. Several varieties of wild garlic grow around the world, usually in wooded areas. Garlic is the most potent of all the alliums, and the most well known for its culinary abilities and its numerous medical applications. The plant is ideally suited to many climates, but prefers to be in a sunny position. Generally, garlic grows best in a light, sandy soil that is not too rich, and its green shoots normally reach up to about three feet high. Beneath the soil lies the bulb, which tends to develop primarily after the plant has flowered. All parts of the plant are scented, but the bulb is the strongest. Each bulb consists of between seven and twenty cloves, which are covered in a papery thin skin. The skin should peel off easily if the garlic is not past its prime. The long pointed leaves are thought to have given rise to the name "gar," meaning in Old English, spear or lance and "leac," meaning leek or pot herb or vegetable.

In Spain the leaves are harvested and form part of a traditional *tapas*. Garlic is best planted in late October or early November to produce a crop the following spring. Later planting in warmer climates, like America, produces a crop in July or August. The flowers are usually small and white, sometimes tinged with green or purple and are densely packed together. Garlic makes a very good companion plant, particularly for roses, who will lose any blackspot when planted near to garlic. It is also said that the roses smell sweeter as they have to manufacture more perfume to overcome their neighbour's special aroma! Other crops thrive as well when garlic is planted nearby, including carrots and leeks. However, because garlic is a plant, its quality will vary, and this depends on the soil nutrient content, relative humidity, sunshine and what is added to or taken away from the soil when cultivated.

Three accepted methods are used for measuring the quality of raw and processed garlic: (1) how much alliin is contained in the garlic bulb also), (2) the total sulphur content, and (3) how microbiologically active the allicin is. Since allicin is the first thing formed when garlic is cut, crushed, cooked, boiled, chopped, stir fried or mechanically processed, scientists have been able to meaure the amount of allicin released from different garlics around the world. The amount of allicin generated from a bulb of garlic can vary by as much as 10 times, but if the growing conditions are favourable, most of the commercially grown garlic (*Allium sativum linn.*) can deliver about a 4% allicin yield.

CHAPTER TWO
A brief chemistry lesson

What does garlic contain?

There are 17 amino acids to be found in garlic: lysine, histidine, arginine, aspartic acid, threonine, serine, glutamine, proline, glycine, alanine, cysteine, valine, methionine, isoleucine, leucine, tryptophan and phenylalanine. Garlic also contains at least 33 sulphur compounds and the minerals germanium, calcium, copper, iron, potassium, magnesium, selenium and zinc; vitamins A, B1 and C, fibre and water, but NO allicin.

The chemistry of Ggarlic—allicin and alliin

In 1944 the chemist Cavallito first isolated an unstable, odourous sulphur-containing compound with antibacterial properties from extracts of fresh garlic. He called this substance allicin (al-e-sin), from the generic name for the plant *Allium Sativum*. In 1948 Stoll and Seebeck discovered the odourless sulphur-containing compound alliin (al-e-een), found in the garlic bulb and enzymatically converted by allinase (al-i-naze), an enzyme found in garlic, when the bulb is crushed.

Analysis of steam distillations of crushed garlic cloves performed over a century ago showed a variety of allyl sulfides. The debate on the presence of allicin in crushed cloves versus its absence in odourless intact cloves was resolved after Stoll and Seebeck isolated, identified, and synthesized an oxygenated sulfur amino acid that is present in large quantities in garlic cloves, which they named *alliin*. This alliin was found to be the stable precursor that is converted to allicin by the action of an enzyme termed *allinase*, also present in the cloves. The transformation of alliin into the biologically-active allicin molecule, upon crushing of a garlic clove, is extremely rapid, completed in seconds. The enzyme responsible for this conversion is allinase, which is present in unusually large amounts in garlic cloves: at least 10% of the total protein content (10 mg/g fresh weight). Garlic cloves are odor-free until cut, crushed, cooked, boiled, chopped, mechanically or chemically processed. Cross-section studies have indicated that the substrate *alliin* and the enzyme *allinase* are located in different compartments of a garlic clove.

This unique organization suggests that it is designed as a potential defense mechanism against microbial pathogens in the soil. Invasion of the cloves by fungi and other soil pathogens causes the interaction between alliin and allinase that rapidly produces allicin, which in turn inactivates the invader. The reactive allicin molecules produced have a very short half-life, since they react with many of the surrounding proteins, including the allinase enzyme, making it into a quasi-suicidal enzyme. This makes it very difficult for allinase to continue reacting with alliin and to form allicin without becoming deactivated.

This very efficient chemical organization ensures that the clove defense mechanism is only activated in a very small location and for a short period of time, whereas the rest of the alliin and allinase remain preserved in their respective compartments and are available for interaction in case of subsequent microbial attacks.

Consequently, this problem has led to the production of a vast number of garlic supplements that are a poor compromise. Either they cannot produce any allicin (because it was destroyed during the manufacture), or they rely on your body to make allicin for you, but this can only happen under ideal conditions without the prescence of stomach acid!

A similar picture is true for the total sulphur content of garlic from around the world, and there is wide variability in the amount of sulphur that can be generated from commercial products. Allicin, however, is only one of the numerous compounds to be produced to varying degrees from all raw garlic. Over the last 20 years, many compounds that are formed from allicin as it degrades have been isolated, characterised and experimented upon. These include isomeric vinyl dithienes and a compound given the name *ajoene* (ah-ho-ene), taken from the Spanish word for garlic, "ajo." These are known as secondary degradation products of alliin. It has been demonstrated in the laboratory that ajoene possesses antithrombotic, antimycotic and fat depositing activities *in vitro* (in the test tube).

The leading authority in the world on garlic chemistry is Professor Block from the State University of New York, and he has determined that ajoene is not found in unprocessed garlic, nor has it ever been isolated from any commercially available garlic supplement until the advent of real allicin found in 100% allicin-yielding products now sold across America.

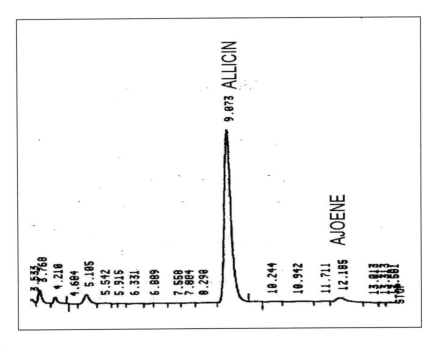

HPLC (high pressure liquid chromatography) trace of allicin liquid produced by Allicin International Limited. This shows one major peak for allicin and a small peak identified as ajoene. The liquid however does not contain alliin or allinase enzyme.

It is reported that, of the 200 or so other sulphur compounds that can be formed when raw garlic is cut or crushed or mechanically disrupted in any way (particularly by boiling), many have not been isolated because they are transitory in nature. Other compounds that have gained scientific interest across a wide spectrum of disease conditions have only been used in experiments on animals or on human cell models. To see an effect with these compounds, the cells may often be transplanted back into host animals.

Thus, allicin is categorised as the "Mother substance" from which all others flow. When raw garlic degrades into allicin to a greater or lesser extent, many "sons and daughters" of allicin will form, some of which may have beneficial effects on the body.

So what is allicin?

Allicin has been variously described as diallyl thiosulphinate, allyl sulphide or even S-(2-Propenyl) 2-propene-1-sulfinothioate. The most crucial and reactive part of the allicin molecule is the sulfur-sulfur bond coupled to the oxygen molecule.

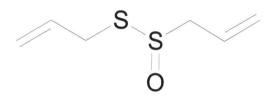

The allicin molecule

This is a very reactive bond which gives allicin (and therefore garlic) its amazing properties as an antibiotic. Before the advent of pharmaceutical antibiotics, crushed garlic extracts were used to treat a wide range of infectious diseases including dysentery, typhus, cholera, smallpox and tuberculosis.

The first class of antibiotics were the sulphonamides, first invented in the 1930s. The reason they were so successful was the prescence of the reactive sulfur group—exactly what allicin contains!

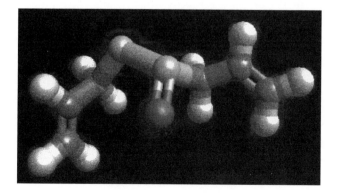

A schematic diagram of the allicin molecule.
Oxford University Department of Chemistry.

Which products can produce allicin?

Allicin yield is determined following conversion to diallyl disulphide. Therefore all commercial products can be assessed for allicin-releasing ability and total sulphur content.

The difference in the proportion of allicin and total sulphur compounds released in various types of garlic, both raw and commercial preparations, is over twentyfold. Therefore, it is important to either buy raw garlic that is rich in alliin (this is of course both impractical and unlikely for consumers today), or to purchase a garlic supplement that has been properly standardized and has not lost the ability to produce a high allicin yield.

Garlic supplements—the good, the bad, and the ugly

For those of us who find it quite impossible to bear the smell or taste of garlic, a wide variety of garlic supplements are available. It can be very confusing, and quite bewildering, when you go into a health food shop or a chemist to purchase a garlic supplement. There are literally hundreds of different brands and lots of "own label" products, all seeming to offer the consumer some healthy allicin!

The independent consumer body, Consumer Labs recent review of garlic supplements *(March 2003)* found strength to vary by as much as 1500% across products. Strength was based on each product's ability to generate allicin in a laboratory test. Consumer Labs found that nearly one-quarter of non-aged products yielded less allicin than generally considered therapeutic.

Garlic is used in the treatment of elevated cholesterol, hypertension, and other diseases. More than 5 million units of garlic were purchased in the past year from drug stores, supermarkets and mass merchandisers in the US. This makes garlic the most popular herbal product according to Information Resources, Inc., and yet NONE of those consumers are getting what they actually need from a garlic product—the allicin.

Thirteen non-aged garlic products and one aged garlic product were purchased and tested by ConsumerLab.com. The amount of allicin produced by the non-aged garlic products ranged from as little as 400 micrograms to 6,500 micrograms per daily recommended serving. Ironically, a product with one of the lowest allicin yields per gram of garlic claimed that it was "Allicin Rich." Another product urged consumers to compare it to a better-known brand that ConsumerLab.com found to yield more than eight times as much allicin. Several products produced nowhere near the amount of allicin they claimed.

"*It is impossible for a consumer to know for sure how strong a garlic product is without testing it,*" said Tod Cooperman, MD, President of ConsumerLab.com. "*Few products clearly state their allicin yield and, when they do, they are not always accurate.*"

The important word in these statements is "yield." This is purely a theoretical yield of allicin, and in reality of the human body, this just does not happen. It is estimated, by garlic experts such as Dr. Larry Lawson and Professor Eric Block, that every time you swallow a garlic powder product, 95% of it will never become active and you will get virtually nothing from it.

A recent paper from the *Journal of Agricultural Food Science* by Lawson and Wang showed that most garlic supplements are standardized on allicin potential and are enteric-coated to prevent gastric acid inactivation of the allicin-producing enzyme allinase. To determine whether these products release the claimed amount of allicin under simulated gastrointestinal conditions (that is the conditions found in YOUR body when you actually swallow these products), USP dissolution method 724A for drug release was applied to all 24 known brands of enteric-coated tablets. It was found that nearly all brands employed effective coatings and that they met their claims for allicin potential when crushed and suspended in water. The researchers went on to say:

"However, all brands except one gave low dissolution allicin release, with 83% of the brands releasing less than 5% of their potential. The low allicin release was found to be due to both impaired allinase activity, mostly caused by tablet excipients, and to slow tablet disintegration, which also impairs allinase activity. Only when tablets had high allinase activity and disintegrated rapidly did they show high allicin release. The ability of USP 724A to estimate allicin release in vivo was validated by monitoring breath levels of the allicin metabolite, allyl methyl sulfide. In conclusion, garlic powder supplements should no longer be standardized on allicin potential, but rather on dissolution allicin release."

Further evidence was published in the same journal by two researchers from The Department of Chemistry at the University of California at Irvine. They analyzed a large number of commercially available garlic products and came to the conclusion that the amount of allicin actually available from these products, when analyzed in gastric or intestinal fluid, would be less than 1ppm. Compare this with a guaranteed 100% yield of at least 300ppm allicin from the new "real allicin-containing" products that we are working with, and you can see that there really is NO comparison.

Oils, pearls, capsules, tablets or raw garlic?

When all is said and done, it is clear that a garlic product that can give you allicin is more likely to improve some of the more serious conditions than one that cannot. With regard to raw garlic, we can show a wide variation in the relative yield of allicin from different garlics around the world and, of course, the social consequences of consuming a lot of garlic are well known to everyone!

Independent analyses carried out at the Camden Food and Drink Research Association and at the universally renowned Warren Springs Laboratory determined the "allicin release" and "total sulphur" content of various commercial preparations. The results reveal that garlic oil, pearl and capsule products are unable to provide allicin because of the method of manufacture. Raw garlic is boiled so that allicin is removed. The resulting sulphur compounds are then concentrated many times so that some oil-based products do contain potentially beneficial sulphur compounds.

Think of it as a family. If you have the mother substance (in this case allicin), then you will get ALL the "sons and daughters" that come from allicin.

Some garlic powder tablet preparations do have the ability to generate tiny quantities of allicin, and therefore all the sulphur compounds that come from allicin will also be present, but the actual amount of allicin that your body receives from these products is minute. This is the main reason why there is absolutely NO DATA published on these products to show any anti-microbial activity. Even recent studies on cardiovascular activity have failed to confirm the promise that earlier studies showed.

Type of Supplement	Fresh garlic source declared on pack supplement	Process to Manufacture	Allicin potential	Published blinded microbial data
Garlic Oil	No	Steam distillation	No	No
Aged Garlic	No	Aged over 2 years	No	No
Garlic Macerates	No	Crushed and dried some		No
Garlic Powder	Sometimes	Cloves chopped and dried under pressure and temperature control	Yes (Stomach acid protection needed)	No
Allicin powder extracts Allisure®	No	Specialised patented extraction process produces allicin liquid that is spray dried product	Product is allicin	Yes

Types of garlic supplement found on health food stores, chemists, drug stores and supermarket shelves

The method of extracting active sulfur chemicals from garlic is also very important. Researchers all over the world have independently shown that when you process garlic and extract, using an oil, you seal up the activity of the sulfur compounds so they will not be readily used by the body. Consequently, the activity against microbial species is severely diminished. Water-based extracts (like real allicin) are MUCH more active. We see such good results against bacterial infections when the "Mother substance" allicin and ALL the other active thiosulphinate substances that allicin breaks down into are available from these water-based extracts.

Chart A highlights the difference by showing that water-based extraction methods are able to kill bacteria even when they are diluted 20-30 times more than oil-based extracts.

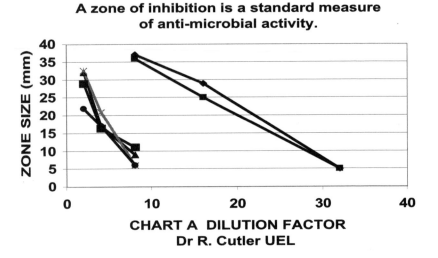

A zone of inhibition is a standard measure of anti-microbial activity.

CHART A DILUTION FACTOR
Dr R. Cutler UEL

Chart B shows the same thing. You can see that the relative concentration of thiosulphinate compounds readily available to your body when extracted from fresh garlic are much greater when you use water as an extraction solvent.

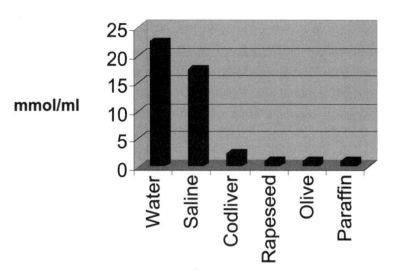

CHART B EXTRACT MEDIUM
Dr R. Cutler UEL

Clearly if you want to produce an extract from fresh garlic that actually works microbiologically, you must use water as an extraction medium. This is the only way of producing a product that can kill bacteria. Liquid allicin is the ultimate extraction process because the alliin in fresh garlic is allowed to completely convert to allicin. The allicin is also removed from the reaction so that it won't interfere with the allinase enzyme that is completing the conversion process.

66Please remember, not all garlic products are created equal, and with the advent of new technology we can now produce and stabilize allicin—the heart of garlic.99

Garlic has the potential to assist the immune system in a number of different ways, stimulating immune cells, killing pathogens and detoxifying carcinogens. Although the compound can be obtained directly from fresh garlic bulbs, one would have to regularly eat very large amounts of cooked garlic to obtain any beneficial effect, and few of us can eat large amounts of raw garlic. This leaves us with liquids and powders. Given the importance of the agent, allicin, any garlic liquids or powders should give an indication of the amount of allicin available from the product, but many do not confirm what happens in the human gut.

Contraindications

Taking too much garlic can quickly prevent blood clotting. People already on anticoagulants, or those about to undergo surgery, should advise their medical team before starting therapy with ANY garlic supplement. Contrary to popular belief, it is not a contraindication. Garlic can also cause reactions in people who are allergic. This is usually mild and will disappear when they stop eating garlic. After surgery, it will usually be sensible to take allicin powder capsules in order to keep your blood thin and vigorously traveling around your circulatory system.

The identity of the active compounds producing effects thus far observed on the immune system with garlic and garlic products is far from conclusive. Since both allicin-derived garlic oils as well garlic extracts not containing allicin are effective *in vivo* at moderate doses, it appears that both allicin and other unidentified compounds are responsible for the effects. Both types of compounds may be important to the overall effects of garlic, since the immune system involves several types of cells, each of which may be affected differently, as has been indicated in the *in vitro* studies.

So please remember, not all garlic products are created equal, but with the advent of new technology, we can now produce and stabilize allicin—the heart of garlic. This means that for the first time anywhere in the world, we have the mother substance from fresh garlic ready, willing and able to get into your body, preventing and treating a wide range of common ailments. The next section details many of the areas where allicin-containing products can really help people.

CHAPTER THREE

A to Z of medical uses

Garlic extracts have been used as medicines for thousands of years, and the spectrum of conditions combatted successfully with this miraculous plant is very wide indeed. Whether or not this activity against common diseases of the day was found by accident, inspiration or simple trial and error, we may never know. But found it was, and quickly garlic established itself as probably the most useful food/medicine in those ancient times. First used for its potent antibiotic properties, it quickly became established as a cleanser of the body, a mild diuretic, a remover of poisons and a healer of wounds and sores. In ancient Egypt, garlic was routinely crushed into water to make an aqueous extract for topical application and ingesting.

Over the centuries, garlic has been used for many things, nearly always with success, and has established a reputation as the "herb all heal." Scientists now agree that allicin is the key to much of garlic's success. An analysis of the medical databases finds over 1500 clinical papers where allicin's activity has been proven. These include:

Proven Pharmacological Activities of Allicin:

Anticoagulation—	thins the blood
Antihypertensive—	reduces blood pressure
Antimicrobial—	kills microscopic organisms

Antibiotic—	kills poisonous bacteria
Antiparasitic—	kills parasites
Antimycotic—	kills fungal infections
Antiviral—	kills viruses
Hypolipidaemic—	reduces high blood cholesterol
Detoxifies heavy metals—	removes lead, mercury and other toxic material
Antitumour—	reduces or prevents cancer tumours
Antioxidant—	scavenges and removes dangerous free radicals
Antiaging—	delays aging
Immune modulator—	repairs the immune system
Humoral immunity—	keeps blood circulation healthy
Fibrinolysis—	reduces blood fibrinogen
Antiplatelet—	reduces blood platelet clumping

It is perhaps worth restating that we have only been able to work with stabilized allicin for a few years, but medical researchers, universities and scientists all over the world have been able to produce small amounts of stabilized allicin by using organic solvents or alcohol to partially stabilize the allicin. Consequently, a huge amount of work has been done to show the wide spectrum of activity attributable to allicin. Only with the advent of a patented extraction method for stabilizing allicin can we now revisit all the areas where we know allicin will be effective. In this section, we look in detail at the variety of conditions that allicin formulations will help.

A to Z of medical uses for allicin

ACNE

Medical definition

Acne vulgaris is a common inflammatory disorder of the sebaceous glands characterized by the presence of blackheads with papules, pustules and in more severe cases, cysts and scars.

Although the actual cause of acne is still unknown, many physicians suggest that it is an infectious disease. The tiny oil-secreting sebaceous glands found in large numbers on the face, upper back and chest may become infected with bacteria. In particular, *Staphylococcus*, *Streptococcus* and *Candida albicans* (a fungus) will accumulate and produce a secondary infection. This leads to a worsening of clinical symptoms, making acne extremely difficult to treat. The major sufferers are teenage adolescents who will do absolutely anything to clean, medicate, cover up or prevent an outbreak. Unfortunately, many antibiotic treatments are unable to kill off *Staphylococcus* infection, since the bacteria are drug resistant! Paying attention to diet is also important, since certain foods can aggravate the condition, especially sugar, caffeine, cocoa, refined vegetable oils as well as various nitrates and sulphites that are used extensively as preservatives in processed foodstuffs.

Allicin powder capsules and allicin liquid are very effective at treating acne for 3 main reasons. Firstly, both formulations routinely kill *Staphylococcus aureus*, *Streptococcus species* and *Candida albicans*. Indeed every batch of these materials that are made are microbiologically tested against a multi-drug-resistant strain of bacteria. Secondly, both allicin formulations are mildly acidic in nature—a big advantage since data suggest that acidic pH is protective and helps to prevent bacterial overgrowth. It is thought that the release of various hormones in the teenage years may contribute toward raising the pH of the skin, so as to attract microbial organisms. Thirdly, allicin liquid is able to dry the skin quickly, which helps to shrink swollen lesions and assist in their removal.

Treatment regimen

It is important to remember that what acne sufferers want is a degree of protection from developing further problems once the disease is under control. It is therefore necessary to get significant allicin into the bloodstream so as to boost the immune system while at the same time, treating the pimples topically with allicin liquid. So take 2-4 capsules every day for at least 4 weeks. At the same time, use a few drops of allicin liquid applied directly to each pimple, and, if you can, add a few more drops to the soap or cleanser that you use each day. Because most people on the planet have already been exposed to garlic, it is unlikely that anyone will be sensitive to any allicin formulation. If this does occur, simply stop the treatment. With regular use of allicin liquid and capsules, significant results can be expected within 2 weeks. At this stage, you can reduce the dose of capsules down to a maintainence dose of just one capsule each day. This is important to remember, since it will help you develop a degree of protection against a further bacterial overgrowth.

AIDS (Acquired immunodeficiency syndrome)
Medical definition

AIDS was first identified in Los Angeles in 1981. A description of the causative virus—the human immunodeficiency virus (HIV)—was available in 1983. The virus destroys a subgroup in lymphocytes, resulting in suppression of the body's immune response. AIDS is essentially a sexually transmitted disease, either homosexually or heterosexually. It is also spread through infected blood, or blood products, and by the mother to her fetus.

For those people who do enter a chronic stage, there may be illness of varying severity, including persistant generalized involvement of the lymph nodes. This is termed ARC (AIDS related complex), with symptoms of intermittent fever, weight loss, diarrhea, fatigue and night sweats. Often opportunistic infections can be life threatening to AIDS sufferers, especially pneumonia caused by the protozoan *(pneumocystis carnii)* and possible tumors leading to Karposi's Sarcoma. It is not actually the HIV virus that kills AIDS patients, but the infections that are easily picked up through a seriously depleted immune system.

Thankfully, large doses of allicin powder can help to prevent infections from developing in HIV and sero-converted AIDS sufferers. By boosting the immune system and destroying a wide range of infectious organisms, allicin powder can definitely help.

In the USA, trials in AIDS patients have demonstrated enhancement of natural killer-cell activity using garlic extracts, and Chinese studies with viral infections in bone marrow transplant patients have demonstrated a "potent antiviral activity." Human population studies have shown that regular intake reduces the risk of esophageal, stomach and colon cancer. This was thought to be due to the antioxidant effect of allicin in reducing the formation of carcinogenic compounds in the gastro-intestinal tract.

"Two days later, I was sitting up, eating a pizza, and enjoying watching television."

Testimonial

David from New York City has been HIV positive for 10 years and has had full-blown AIDS for 2 years. He picked up a serious infection and used large doses of allicin powder capsules to get rid of this infection.

He said *"I can attest to the strength and promise of allicin powder capsules. For a quick example, I was experiencing diarrhea about once every day or two—and then I started taking the capsules. Since I started using them, I have not had diarrhea ONCE. I have been using Allisure® powder for about two months now.*

"More dramatically, when I received my first shipment in the mail, I

had been sick for three days with a viral infection and had been feeling worse each day. On the third day, I was really quite miserable and ill, especially realizing this illness could go on for two or three weeks—or worse. I started taking my first capsule toward the end of that third day, and two days later (Superbowl Sunday evening in the US), I was sitting up, eating a pizza, and enjoying watching television. I was surprised that I felt so much better in such a relatively short (48 hours) period of time. By the end of the third day, I felt like I was basically over my viral infection, and that the "bug" had been killed. Naturally, I was not back to full vigor just yet, but each day, on Allisure capsules, I felt stronger, healthier and more vigorous. I was back to my full strength and vigor in about ten days, which is about what it would be for anyone. I was astounded at the healing power that allicin apparently contains. I feel like allicin will, in time, prove itself to be essentially an "immune system in pill form," seemingly without any drawbacks, side-effects, etc. The potential for improved health for humankind could—based on my own personal experience—be enormous, truly staggering.

"I consider allicin powder capsules to be a medical miracle."

"If allicin could offer this kind of powerful help to someone in my condition, what could it do for people with normal immune systems? Since I've started using this product, I have not experienced any other abnormal health problems at all, and I'm not taking any other medicines. I'm now beginning to think that I may be able to "get my life back," return to work, etc. This as opposed to thinking that my days were more or less 'numbered'! I now once again do things that I enjoy—with confidence—for I no longer feel afraid to over-exert myself physically, etc. My life has, relatively speaking, 'gone back to normal.'

I consider allicin powder capsules to be a medical miracle."

Then a few weeks later David sent me another letter:

"More good news—after years of having 'borderline-high' blood pressure, my last visit to the doctor tells me my blood pressure is 'good'! At first I thought, 'How could that be possible? Why would my blood pressure suddenly be so different?' I think it's the allicin. I can't think of any other change in my life that might have lowered my blood pressure to such a degree."

ANIMAL BITES

Animal bites are very common with over 2 million Americans bitten by dogs each year. Wildlife animal bites and human bites also cause a significant number of trips to the ER as well. A bite of any description can be immediately very painful and, with an open wound, the passage of infectious organisms is simple.

Usually a bite from an animal can be deep into the flesh, which means that it is very easy for microbes to get directly into the blood and surrounding tissue. Because of this, many physicians refuse to suture an animal bite, since this would effectively seal in the infection. Consequently, this leads to poor wound healing as well as a potentially life-threatening infection. History records that many serious global infections have been easily transferred from the animal population to humans.

In this situation, allicin formulations have a major role to play in preventing the passage of infection. Allicin liquid has the capability to kill a wide range of invasive organisms. By backing liquid allicin up with a regular course of allicin capsules, infection from animal bites can be prevented.

Treatment regimen

After washing the wound thoroughly, squeeze in a few drops of allicin liquid. This may sting a little, but don't be afraid to persevere. Repeat 2-3 times a day for at least a week. The wound should begin to heal quickly. At the same time, take 2-3 allicin powder capsules daily for a period of about 6 weeks to make sure you have sufficient allicin in your bloodstream to remove any pathogens that may be present. This was how one of my relatives approached a nasty dog bite.

ARTHRITIS
With ginger
Medical definition

Although arthritis literally means "joint inflammation," anyone who has one of the many forms of arthritis and related conditions knows the condition often extends far beyond bones and cartilage, including Sjögren's syndrome, psoriasis and irritable bowel syndrome. By some estimates, as many as 70 percent of people with fibromyalgia have symptoms of irritable bowel syndrome (IBS)—abdominal pain and bloating along with constipation or diarrhea or alternating bouts of the two.

For thousands of years, garlic extracts have been used to heal the pain and inflammation of arthritis. In the Middle Ages it was common practice, recommended by herbalists, to crush fresh garlic into a piece of muslin and wrap the cloth around an arthritic joint. This eased the pain and helped to reduce the swelling. Allicin, when combined with ginger, is an ideal combination to take orally to help ease the misery of rheumatoid arthritis.

Treatment regimen

Take 2 allicin capsules with ginger 3 times a day, either in addition to current medication or alone. The active ingredients will quickly be absorbed into the joints and help to improve mobility. This is a treatment that needs to be continued long-term.

ASTHMA

Medical definition

Widespread narrowing of the bronchial airways, which can change in severity over short periods of time. Symptoms include coughing, sneezing and shortness of breath. Asthma is caused by a wide range of allergens in the air, drug reactions from, aspirin and other non-steroidal anti-inflammatory agents, beta-blockers, or excessive exertion, infections or stressful emotion.

In the United States and Great Britain, the incidence of asthma has reached almost epidemic levels. Not only are the death rates increasing, but there appears to be no respite as we consistently challenge our bodies with poor diet, environmental toxins, and excessive use of drugs. Now that we are constantly under threat from bacterial and viral attacks, simple infections like the common cold, coughs and sore throats can trigger an asthma attack. Yet we have also known for thousands of years that garlic can help to vasodilate the bronchial airways. And now we also know that allicin can prevent and treat the common cold, coughs, sore throats and a wide range of bacterial, viral and fungal disease than can trigger the classic asthma symptoms.

Treatment regimen

Take 1 to 4 allicin powder capsules every day and double this dose at times when you can predict the onset of asthma attack.

ATHLETE'S FOOT

Medical definition

*This is a fungal infection of the skin, the scalp or the nails, caused by the dermatophyte fungi—*Trichopyton *and* Epidermatophyton. *This can also affect animals, which is often a source of infection for man.*

The fungus can be spread by direct contact or via infected materials. The lesions are often ring-like and may cause intense itching. The most common form is athlete's foot, which affects the skin between the toes.

Another common type is ringworm of the scalp *(tinea capitis)*, a severe form. Ringworm also affects the groin and thighs *(tinea cruris)*, also known as jock itch, and even the skin under a beard can become infected *(tinea barbae)*.

Of all the species that are killed by various allicin formulations, it is the fungal organisms that appear to be the most sensitive—that is, they are the easiest to kill. Research reports that allicin is effective *in vitro* against species of *Candida, Cryptococcus, Trichophyton, Epidermphyton* and *Microsporum* at low concentration. Allicin inhibits both germination of spores and growth of hyphae. The mode of action of allicin on the fungal cell has not yet been determined but it is assumed to function on thiol enzymes as in other microorganisms.

"I find the capsules are easy to take and do not make me smell!"

Treatment regimen

Treatment with allicin liquid or creme is very easy. Just apply one or two drops of liquid between the toes or simply cover with creme. This should be done twice daily for approximately 4 to 6 weeks. Within a few hours, the itchiness will subside. If it returns, then another application should be made. For faster results, use the more concentrated liquid. Once the cracking has begun to heal, start on the capsules to act as a prevention against recurrent infection.

Testimonial

Mr. KL from Birmingham, Alabama, says he started using the liquid as a treatment for athlete's foot back in February 2002 and continues to take allicin powder capsules each day. "The results are different to those of other treatments in that it does not dry out the skin but kills the infected tissue. Therefore, the incidence of cracking between the toes is virtually eliminated. The overall time scale is slightly slower than pharmaceutical drugs, but it certainly keeps the complaint at bay. Interestingly, it has not returned in over 9 months, which is very unusual since I often get recurrent infections. I find the capsules are easy to take and do not make me smell!"

BACTERIAL INFECTIONS

Medical definition

A group of microorganisms all of which lack a distinct nuclear membrane and are considered to be more primitive than animal, plant or human cells. Most bacteria are single-celled and may comprise the following shapes:

- Spherical—*Coccus*
- Rod shaped—*Bacillus*
- Spiral—*Spirillium*
- Comma shaped—*Vibrio*
- Corkscrew shaped—*Spirochete*

Bacteria reproduce asexually by a simple division of cells and an incomplete separation of daughter cells can lead to the formation of colonies consisting of different numbers and arrangements of cells all with different and complex shapes. Bacteria are very widely distributed. Some live in soil, water or air; others are parasites of man, animals and plants and many cause disease by producing toxins.

Antibacterial activity of allicin

The antibacterial properties of crushed garlic have been known for a long time. Various water-based garlic preparations have been shown to exhibit a wide spectrum of antibacterial activity against Gram-negative and Gram-positive bacteria including species of *Escherichia*, *Salmonella*, *Staphylococcus*, *Streptococcus*, *Klebsiella*, *Proteus*, *Bacillus*, *and Clostridium*. Even acid-fast bacteria, such as *Mycobacterium tuberculosis*, are sensitive to allicin, as is *Helicobacter pylori*, often deemed as the the cause of gastric ulcers. Allicin extracts can also prevent the formation of *Staphylococcus* enterotoxins A, B, and C1 and also thermonuclease. Allicin is the only antibiotic that can actually kill infecting bacteria, and at the same time protect the body from the poisons that are causing the infection. It is known that the most sensitive bacterium to allicin is the deadly *Bacillus anthracis*, which produces the poison anthrax.

Cavalito and Bailey were the first to demonstrate that the antibacterial action of garlic is mainly due to allicin. The sensitivity of various bacterial and clinical isolates to pure preparations of allicin is very significant. As shown in the table below the antibacterial effect of allicin is of a broad spectrum. In most cases the 50% lethal dose concentrations were somewhat higher than those required for some of the newer antibiotics. Interestingly, various bacterial strains resistant to antibiotics such as methicillin resistant *Staphylococcus aureus* as well as other multidrug-resistant enterotoxicogenic strains of *Escherichia coli*, *Enterococcus*, *Shigella dysenteriae*, *Shigella flexneni*, and *Shigella sonnei* cells were all found to be sensitive to allicin.

Bacterial Strain	Allicin Concentration (LD50 µg/ml) [# of allicin capsules to take each day to remove the infection]		Comments
Escherichia coli	15	[6]	Sensitive to antibiotics
Escherichia coli	15	[6]	Multidrug resistant MDR
Staphylococcus aureus	12	[5]	Sensitive
Staphylococcus aureus	12	[5]	Methicillin resistant
Streptococcus pyogenes	3	[2]	Sensitive
Streptococcus A hemolyticus	>100	[12]	Clinical MDR strain
Proteus mirabilis	15	[6]	Sensitive
Proteus mirabilis	>30	[8]	Clinical MDR strain
Pseudomonas aeruginosa	15	[6]	Sensitive to cefprozil
Pseudomonas aeruginosa	>100	[12]	MDR mucoid strain
Acinetobacter baumanii	15	[5]	Clinical isolate
Klebsiella pneumoniae	8	[3]	Clinical isolate

Bacterial species' sensitivity to aqueous garlic extracts containing allicin

Most recently the University of East London has shown that aqueous extracts of allicin, when formulated into a simple cream, are able to kill vast swaths of the so-called "superbug" MRSA (methicillin-resistant *Staphylococcus aureus*). This nasty bacterium is forever changing its structure and developing resistance to many pharmaceutical antibiotics. Allicin cream may have a beneficial effect on people who suffer from skin diseases such as eczema and acne, since this bacterium is much more likely to colonize in these patients.

The antibacterial properties of crushed garlic have been known for many years, and a wide variety of extraction methods have been utilized by researchers around the world to produce a garlic extract that can be shown to kill bacterial species. Aqueous (water) extracts are much more active than oil-based extracts (see Chapter 2). Activity can be demonstrated against a wide spectrum of bacteria including species of *Escherichia*, *Salmonella*, *Staphylococcus*, *Streptococcus*, *Klebsiella*, *Proteus*, *Bacillus*, and *Clostridium*. Even acid-fast bacteria such as *Mycobacterium tuberculosis* are sensitive (see Tuberculosis data).

Allicin is also effective against *Helicobacter pylori*, the cause of gastric ulcers. Allicin formulations can also prevent the formation of *Staphylococcus enterotoxins*.

Even bacterial strains such as the mucoid strains of *Pseudomonas aeruginosa*, *Streptococcus β hemolyticus* and *Enterococcus faecium*, were found to be sensitive to the action of allicin, but were concentration dependent. This is very exciting since these organisms have developed hydrophilic capsular or mucoid layers to prevent the penetration of antimicrobial agents.

The minimum inhibitory concentration of allicin in parts per million for some common bacterial species:

Streptococcus pyogenes	16 ppm	(flesh eating bacteria)
Staphylococcus aureus	16 ppm	(nosocomial infection)
Listeria monocytogenes	16 ppm	(often caught from animals)
Escherichia Coli 0157	32 ppm	(poorly cooked meat)
Salmonella typhimurium	32 ppm	(raw eggs)
Clostridium perfringens	64 ppm	(animals and man)
Helicobacter pylori	16 ppm	(stomach ulcers)
Yersinia enterocolitica	12 ppm	(stomach upsets)
Bacillus subtilus	<3 ppm	(causes conjunctivitis)

Now at last we have REAL STABILISED ALLICIN to work with and, in a short period of time, we have seen that allicin has the ability to kill a wide range of drug-resistant bacteria. In every country where allicin powder capsules, creme or liquid are available, drug-resistant bacterial infections have been cured!

Drug-resistant *Streptococcus*

In the country of Norway a young mother of 2 children went into the hospital for her third child. She was due to have a Cesarian section and everything went according to plan and a baby boy was born. Unfortunately, Camilla picked up an infection. This is common, not just in Norway, but in just about every country in the world. Camilla had a drug-resistant streptococcus, and after being discharged from the hospital, her wound failed to heal for several months. She had a systemic infection that made her tired, washed out and unable to look after her new baby or the family. Things got worse, so much so that her husband had to take time off work to look after her and the family. Camilla was given successive courses of antibiotics, but for months and months she could not get rid of the infection.

"No bacteria found in her throat, her underarms or her vagina. She was clear, healthy and happy!"

Camilla was desperate! She was ill and couldn't bond with her new baby. Then one day she read in her newspaper about a new product that kills bacteria—a natural plant extract that came from fresh garlic called Weissin (the name chosen in Norway for allicin powder products). She contacted the supplier and they told her how to get the product. Camilla took 10 capsules per day, every day for 4 weeks, and to her delight she began to feel better. She had already stopped taking the antibiotics, and in less than a month, the regular specimens she had to provide for the hospital came back negative—no bacterial infection. No bacteria was found in her throat, her underarms or her vagina. She was clear, healthy and very happy!

The allicin had completely destroyed a multi-drug-resistant Streptococcal bacterial infection. Camilla was happy and able to bond with her new baby for the first time since he was born. Her husband was able to return to work and life could at last return to normal.

BAD BREATH

The dreaded "garlic breath" is usually what deters people from eating large quantities of fresh or cooked garlic. Consequently, many people have quite rightly turned to supplements to obtain the benefits without the social side effects! However, as we learned earlier in this book, the most common reason why people stop taking a garlic supplement is because they smell! It is usually a casual observation made by a partner, friend or child, asking, "What have you been eating?"

This is never a problem with allicin supplements, because the active allicin is quickly absorbed and will get into the bloodstream unnoticed. Remember to take the allicin capsules with a little cool liquid and preferably with your main meal. Sometimes if you take a large dose you may notice the allicin, but this will only last for a few minutes and will not continue to regurgitate on your breath. It may even be beneficial in this respect if you suffer from sinusitis or rhinitis, since the allicin will reflux back up into your nasal cavity and get to work immediately.

BED SORES

Medical definition

An ulcerated area of skin caused by irritation and constant pressure on a part of the body. Healing is prevented by a decreased blood supply, and the formation of gangrene must be avoided.

This is an exciting area of research with allicin, since garlic has two important functions with regard to healing wounds (see later section on wound healing). Not only can you expect to start healing faster if you apply allicin liquid to the pressure bandage, but you will prevent an infection from developing. Research is currently underway in this area.

BLADDER INFECTIONS—Cystitis
Medical definition

This is an inflammation of the urinary bladder usually caused by Escherichia coli. It is usually accompanied by the desire to pass urine frequently and with a degree of burning. A severe infection usually causes a persistent, cramplike pain in the lower abdomen.

Allicin capsules will certainly get to the root cause of the problem—the bacterial infection. We live in a world where antibiotics are overused and misused. This has led to the development of a large number of drug-resistant strains of bacteria that are extremely difficult to eradicate. This situation can also lead to a secondary fungal infection that can be present in the bladder, urethra, vagina and even the kidneys. Because allicin has such a wide spectrum of activity and because results demonstrate effectiveness in killing drug-resistant bacteria, allicin capsules will be worthwhile using for ANY microbial infection.

Incredibly, allicin can kill *E.coli* at a concentration of just 16ppm, and we have even seen activity against the deadly strain *E. coli 0157* at just 32ppm.

Treatment regimen

Take 3-6 allicin capsules every day for at least 4 weeks. Any vaginal irritation can be treated with allicin liquid by placing 10 drops into plain yogurt and inserting in the vagina.

BLOOD PRESSURE
Medical definition

The pressure of the blood against the walls of the arteries. Pressure is highest during systole when the heart ventricles are contracting (systolic pressure) and lowest during diastole, when the ventricles are relaxing and refilling. The normal range of blood pressure varies and increases with age. A young adult would be expected to have a blood pressure of 120/80 (systolic/diastolic).

High blood pressure is described as a "silent killer," because it can creep up on you and strike, without causing symptoms, to trigger a sudden heart attack or stroke. Even if your blood pressure is very high, you may feel relatively well without showing any obvious signs or symptoms. Some people with high blood pressure may feel dizzy and develop a headache. It is therefore important to ensure that levels are kept as near to normal as possible.

Blood pressure varies considerably throughout the day as a result of both physical activity and stress. Usually your blood pressure is at its lowest in the middle of the night and tends to rise to a peak at about 11 A.M. Physical exercise will cause a temporary rise in blood pressure, which is entirely normal, but people with hypertension will have a high blood pressure reading even while resting. Factors that increase the risk of developing high blood pressure are similar to those linked to coronary heart disease and include increasing age, smoking cigarettes, obesity, excess alcohol intake, a family history of heart disease, lack of exercise and high stress levels.

It is estimated by medical experts that by reducing your diastolic blood pressure by as little as 5 mmHg would decrease the risk of developing coronary heart disease by a massive 16 per cent. Allicin can do much more than this!

There are many prescription drugs available to reduce blood pressure. While they are very effective, they can cause side-effects. Allicin has now been shown to significantly reduce both systolic and diastolic blood pressure. Only recently the prestigious medical journal *The Journal of Hypertension* reported that garlic extracts with an available allicin yield of just 0.6% could reduce systolic blood pressure by 10 percent and diastolic blood pressure by 6 percent. The journal went on to say that the potential blood pressure lowering effect of this natural plant medicine was of such significance "**that stroke may be reduced by 30 to 40 percent and coronary heart disease by 20 to 25 percent.**"

Now we have a product range with an available allicin yield of 100%, so we would expect to see both systolic and diastolic blood pressure lowered by at least 10%. Applying these results to the general population, we could expect to reduce the incidence of coronary heart disease by 25 percent, which could mean at least 145,000 lives saved each and every year by allicin in the USA alone.

A modern-day epidemic

In 1969 the executive board of the World Health Organization reported that "Coronary heart disease has reached enormous proportions, striking more and more at younger subjects. It will result in coming years in the greatest epidemic mankind has faced unless we are able to reverse this trend by concentrated research into its cause and prevention."

Coronary heart disease is the number one killer in the developed world and the most common cause of death in the UK. Upon examination of the league table of deaths from coronary heart disease (CHD) in different countries, Scotland and Northern Ireland rank at the top, only surpassed in the total number of deaths by Finland. In England and Wales there has been a reduction in deaths over recent years, but much work still needs to be done.

In the UK alone, around 170,000 people die from a heart attack every year—nearly 500 a day. Considering that we now have over 2 million angina sufferers and approximately 20 per cent of the adult population has high blood pressure, the majority of our entire population also has a raised level of blood cholesterol. The level of obesity continues to grow, our average amount of useful exercise continues to shrink, the incidence of sugar diabetes continues to rise, and our national diet is derided almost every day in the press and media! Thus you begin to see that we have a lot of work to do to reduce the terrible burden this disease puts upon our society.

How does allicin work?

The mechanism of allicin's action on blood pressure is not fully understood, however, it does appear to act as a vasodilator. Studies suggest that allicin powder capsules may exert an ability to lower blood pressure by acting like prostaglandin E_1, which decreases peripheral vascular resistance. What is clear is that to get any significant effect, you must be able to get the active ingredient allicin released into your circulatory system. Most garlic oil, capsules and pearl preparations are not able to provide any allicin, consequently they have no research studies on blood pressure effects.

Treatment regimen

Studies are currently underway to determine the most effective dose of allicin powder capsules for the treatment of blood pressure. We have seen a large number of excellent testimonial statements from people who have seen a significant drop in both systolic and diastolic blood pressure while taking allicin. It is currently recommended that you take between 1 and 6 capsules a day, depending on your current blood pressure reading. Those on medication need not worry, since allicin powder capsule products can be added into ANY blood pressure medication. There may even be a synergistic activity meaning that you should be able to, under supervision from your physician, reduce the dose of medication that you take.

Testimonial

Mr. Steve B from High Wycombe in the UK writes:

"Dear Peter, Just a note to let you know that I have been able to stop taking the beta-blocker drug that was causing me so many problems and not really controlling my blood pressure. As you suggested I started taking 4 allicin capsules a day and monitoring my blood pressure reading. After 6 weeks I persuaded my GP to take me off the drug as I was having some personal problems with it! He took my blood pressure again 2 weeks later (whilst only taking the allicin) and to our combined delight my blood pressure was basically normal. I have kept taking the capsules you sent me but reduced the dose down to 2 per day and my last BP reading was still normal. Thank you so very much for your help."

BOILS

Allicin liquid added to olive oil or apple cider vinegar, made into a lint dressing and applied to the area affected and changed every day, will quickly reduce inflammation and ease pain associated with boils and cysts.

CANDIDIASIS

Medical definition

This is a common yeast infection found in moist areas of the body. It is especially common in the vagina where it is known as thrush, but it is also found in the mouth and skin folds. On the skin the lesions are bright red with small satellite pustules, while in the mouth it appears as white patches on the tongue or inside the cheeks. In the vagina it can produce intense itching and sometimes a thick white discharge. Candida infection can sometimes develop in people who are taking antibiotics or have a poorly-functioning immune system. *Candida albicans* is often now resistant to a wide range of pharmaceutical antifungal agents.

The form we call thrush is associated with the overgrowth of the yeast *candida albicans*. Approximately one in five women carries this yeast in low levels, but it can get out of control if anything happens to disrupt the body's defences.

This could be caused by:
- Stress
- Low immunity
- Hormonal changes around the menstrual period
- The contraceptive pill
- Pregnancy
- Diabetes
- Sex with an infected partner

Symptoms can include:
- Intense itching of the vagina/vulva
- Constant tiredness
- Muscular aches and pains
- Mood swings
- Thick/white discharge
- With oral thrush, white patches in the throat
- Digestive problems

Facts and figures

Up to 10 million women and five million men in the UK are affected by candida. Around 70 million women and 30 million men in the USA will be affected by candida. At least three out of four women will experience thrush at some time in their lives. Symptoms of thrush can include muscular aches, mood swings, drowsiness, recurrent cystitis and severe itching. Caused by the yeast *candida albicans*, thrush is one of the most common forms of vaginal infection.

Antifungal activity of allicin

Garlic extracts also have a strong antifungal effect and inhibit the formation of mycotoxins like the aflatoxin of *Aspergillus parasiticus*. Allicin was assumed to be the main component responsible for the inhibition of fungal growth. In addition, *in vitro* synergistic fungistatic activity with amphotericin B was demonstrated against all isolates of *Cryptococcus neoformans*. Allicin liquid was found to have a high anticandidal activity with a very low minimum inhibitory concentration needed to destroy the fungus. Allicin inhibits both germination of spores and growth of hyphae. The sensitivities of various clinically important yeasts to a pure preparation of allicin were determined and found to be very significant (see table). The mode of action of allicin on the fungal cell has not yet been elucidated, but it is assumed to function on thiol enzymes as in other microorganisms.

Fungal strain	Allicin concentration MIC ppm allicin	Comments
Candida albicans	1.7ppm	
Candida albicans	4.0 ppm	Clinical isolates
Candida neoformans	1.7 ppm	Drug resistant
Candida parapsilosis	1.4 ppm	
Candida tropicalis	1.7 ppm	
Candida krusei	1.7 ppm	Drug resistant
Torulopsis glabrata	1.7 ppm	

Effect of allicin on various fungal pathogens

Treatment regimen

Begin by taking at least 3-6 capsules of allicin powder every day, taken all at once or throughout the day. This will need to be continued for approximately 1 month, depending on how deep-seated the yeast infection is in your body.

If you have a vaginal discharge, try adding a few drops of allicin liquid to plain yogurt and take orally once or twice a day, again for about 1 month. This will have a cooling and soothing effect and should help to remove the itchiness that is so frustrating for many sufferers. Once progress has been made, it is important to keep to a healthy diet free from excessive sugar and continue taking a daily dose of just 1 or 2 allicin powder capsules. This will help prevent the infection from returning.

Testimonial use

Thrush is the most common form of candida, affecting three out of four women in the UK and eight out ten women in the USA at some time in their lives. One woman tells us what living with candida is really like, and shares advice on managing the condition.

American, Jane Jones, 35, lives in Kent, England and has struggled to manage recurring candida infections since her teens. She reports:

"The first time I got thrush I was only 15 and had no idea what it was. I had a white vaginal discharge and terrible itching. I thought it must be something to do with my periods, or that I'd caught something from a toilet seat. I kept it to myself for a few months until it became really bad. I finally broke down in tears and told my mum, who took me to a male gynaecologist. It was an awful experience. He seemed to think I was sexually active—which I wasn't. It made me feel dirty. As I now know, although thrush can be transferred to a sexual partner, it's not necessarily caused by sex but by an overgrowth of the candida fungus in the system.

"After that first time, the thrush kept on coming back. My mum took me to a couple of female doctors who prescribed the same standard medication, which was Monostat 7 (I was living in America at the time). This was effective at first, but I think I became immune after a while, as I had to take it so often. The doctors also gave me the same advice: don't wear tight jeans, tights or synthetic underwear, avoid perfumed bathing products that can irritate the vagina and always use protection if you are sexually active. The treatments were very focused on the vagina and on curing the symptoms. Nobody ever mentioned dealing with candida throughout the entire body.

"At this time of my life I was so unhappy that I let the candida get me down."

"A few years later, many of the medications I was using became available over the counter so I didn't have to keep going to the doctor, and it became easier to self-treat the condition. But the thrush still kept coming back, so I never felt free of it. I remember getting it badly when I was at university. The discomfort and itching were sometimes so severe I thought I'd go mad. I used to scratch myself until it hurt, because the pain was better than the itching. I didn't confide in anyone about it. In a way I tried to pretend it wasn't there. I was shy around boys, and the boys didn't help my confidence. Whenever I had an outbreak, I felt embarrassed and ashamed, even though there was nothing to be ashamed of. But psychologically it does get you down. You start to feel as if it's somehow your fault.

"After university, I went to live in London and then got married. During this time I started to feel generally tired and unwell. I was still having thrush all the time, but didn't relate the two. My doctor thought I might have glandular fever. I was reading up on the subject at the time and learned that candida overgrowth can have more widespread effects on the system, from bloating to chronic fatigue and digestive problems. I started to think that maybe I didn't simply have vaginal thrush; perhaps there was something going on in my whole body. I realised that when the candida is really bad I don't just have thrush—I feel ill, tired and slow, like I can't think straight. One of the worst things is having no energy. I'm usually quite energetic, so feeling so tired for much of the time is very frustrating.

"At this time of my life I was so unhappy that I let the candida get me down. It was as though thrush was taking over my body, and I didn't feel like myself any more. I also thought the treatment I'd been having was simply addressing the symptoms of the problem rather than the root causes, and that's why it kept coming back.

"I decided to consult a nutritional therapist, who suggested I follow a strict anti-yeast diet. I was advised to avoid all fungi and products with fermented ingredients, such as bread, cheese and alcohol. At the same time, I was also taking a probiotic supplement, acidophilus, to help maintain my body's "good" bacteria and keep the candida in check, and natural supplements such as garlic. My diet was something that I knew I could control and it was great to be able to do something practical, even though it was quite hard to stick to. I had to cut out all sugar, which feeds the fungi, so even seemingly "healthy" food such as fruit was out, as well as things you wouldn't think of, such as peanuts, since they contain a naturally occurring fungus.

"I followed the diet for three months and it helped tremendously. I was symptom-free for about four years. Over that period, I gradually returned to eating normally—enjoying fruit, chocolate and sugary foods. I continued taking acidophilus tablets regularly, but I almost forgot about the candida. Then, about two years ago, I went through a stressful time, took two courses of antibiotics and within a couple of months, started to get thrush again. (I now know it can also be associated with stress, low immunity and using antibiotics, which can disrupt the balance of natural flora in the body.) I used Canesten cream and pessaries or Diflucan tablets and it cleared up. But it started to come back more regularly and became so frequent that I went to my GP to check if my symptoms weren't connected to anything more serious.

"I was tested for diabetes and liver disease, which can both be characterised by recurrent thrush, but fortunately I didn't have either. I cut fruit and sugary foods from my diet again and started taking allicin powder capsules and vitamin C. I'd read about the curative anti-fungal properties of allicin in a book on garlic and found out that *Candida albicans* was one of the most sensitive species. I started on 6 capsules a day for about 4 weeks. At the same time, I even tried aromatherapy, which is quite controversial as the treatment involves douching with essential oils, and thrush sufferers are normally advised to avoid anything that may cause irritation. But I felt I had nothing to lose. Everything I've tried has had some kind of positive effect, though nothing has managed to keep candida away for good until recently. It has now been 12 months since I started on allicin capsules, and I now take just one a day. This seems to prevent the infection from returning. My life is now much more settled, and I feel fit and healthy for the first time in years."

A second testimonial

"Allisure is quite good when sprinkled on toast or over a salad. This product has a big benefit for those who suffer from fungal infestation. Because candida is dimorphic, it can be stubborn to eradicate. My experience with Allisure has been one of great benefit for my staff. When using the Allisure on a consistent basis, dozens of my staff have eliminated stubborn problems with sinus and colds/flu." Lorin Dyrr, Executive Vice President, Global Health Trax

CANKER SORES

Canker sores are a sign of poor immunity and they can often develop as a reaction to toxic elements found in a variety of common foodstuffs. Canker sores usually occur in the mouth and are extremely painful. They are often difficult to treat and tend to heal rather slowly. Most doctors now believe that they are caused by a Streptococcus bacteria which is capable of ulcerating mucous membranes.

Treatment regimen

Dissolve 2 allicin powder capsules in a little water and then gargle for approximately 1 minute. Repeat this every hour for about 4 hours, then repeat each day. You should immediately gain some pain relief, and within 1 week your sore should have healed. Then continue to take 1 capsule daily for maintainence.

CELLULITIS
Medical definition
Cellulitis is defined as large-scale inflammation and infection of the connective tissue between adjacent tissues and organs. This is commonly due to bacterial infection by streptococci species and occasionally by staphylococci species.

It is important to stop the infection spreading to the bloodstream, since this can lead to serious problems that could require hospitalization.

Treatment regimen
If the infection is mild and manifests itself topically, apply a few drops of allicin liquid to each abrasion, twice daily. Supplement this treatment by taking at least 4 allicin powder capsules daily and continue this regimen for 14 days.

If you have a long-term infection that has not been touched by successive courses of antibiotics, it is important to double the dose of allicin powder capsules and stay on this increased dose for at least 3 months. When there is a sign of any improvement, it would be possible to reduce the dose to 1-2 capsules a day.

CHOLESTEROL CONTROL
Medical definition
A fatty-like material present in the blood and in most tissues. Cholesterol is an important constituent of cell membranes and is the precursor to many steroid hormones and bile salts. Western dietary intake of cholesterol is approximately 500-1000mg per day.

Cholesterol is synthesized in the body from acetate, mainly in the liver, and blood concentration should be between 100-300mg/dL Elevated levels of cholesterol are associated with atheroma and need to be controlled.

Cholesterol and lipid-lowering effects of garlic
We now know from long-term epidemiological studies (population studies where the characteristics of an entire population are scrutinised

in considerable detail) that the incidence of coronary heart disease is lowest where the most garlic is eaten. The Italians, Greeks, Spanish, and the populations of Asia and China all have much lower rates of coronary heart disease, and all eat much more garlic than we do in the UK (or America for that matter).

While this is not the complete picture, let us examine one particular study that looked at three groups of vegetarians called the Jains from India. Three groups of diet-matched subjects were investigated and categorised as follows: Group 1 ate more than 50g of garlic and onion per week in their diets and had done so consistently; Group 2 ate no more than 10g of garlic or onion per week and, Group 3 was forbidden to eat any garlic or onion on religious grounds.

When an analysis of their blood cholesterols was conducted, group 1 (lots of garlic) had the lowest cholesterol levels at 175 mg/dL. Group 2 (moderate levels of garlic) had moderate levels of cholesterol at 200 mg/dL and, Group 3 (no garlic) had the highest levels of cholesterol at 250 mg/dL.

Clearly, something in garlic is helping to lower cholesterol levels of entire poulations. Medical studies have also managed to confirm a wide range of other "risk factors" that contribute to the development of a raised cholesterol.

Risk factors

The major risk factors for coronary heart disease are well known:
- increasing age
- eating too much saturated fat
- having a family history of heart disease
- being a male (or a post-menopausal woman)
- poorly controlled insulin diabetes
- drinking excessive amounts of alcohol
- high stress levels
- uncontrolled high blood pressure

- raised blood fat levels
- smoking cigarettes
- being overweight or obese
- insufficient exercise
- visiting a physician who likes prescribing pharmaceutical drugs!

That last point is a little facetious, but in today's world physicians are constantly pressurized into prescribing drugs to everyone who has a cholesterol level over 200 mg/dL. Even the author (a diabetic of 35 years standing) has been counselled by his physician on the need to consider taking an HMGCoA (reductase inhibitor) for the rest of my life to protect my cholesterol level—which by the way is perfectly normal!

Of course some of these risk factors we can do nothing about, and some are either very difficult to change or seemingly impossible to live without! Some we CAN help by making a few simple alterations to our lifestyle. The first step is to start taking allicin powder capsules!

Allicin and cholesterol reduction

It is now known and accepted throughout the world that an increased cholesterol level raises your risk of developing heart disease. High cholesterol is another major risk factor for the development of coronary heart disease. There are two types of circulating cholesterol. One is protective, and the other is known to cause heart disease. Blood fats or lipids, as they are often known, are transported in our bodies by carriers known as lipoproteins. The helpful cholesterol is known as HDL or high-density lipoprotein, which is a large molecule. The other type of cholesterol is harmful, known as LDL or low-density lipoprotein, which is a much smaller molecule.

Usually LDL cholesterol can become oxidized, and this leads to the deposition of harmful fats into the coronary arteries surrounding the heart. It is this build up of fat that can lead to a narrowing of the important coronary arteries. This can then lead to a heart attack, where blood flow is stopped, or to a stroke where a blood clot is dislodged and travels to the heart or brain.

Clearly, anything that we can do to reduce the levels of this harmful fat in our systems will relieve the pressure on our heart and circulatory system.

Throughout the 1980s and 1990s, a number of studies on various garlic supplements were published around the world. Researchers felt these studies were not very well put together, but they all seemed to suggest a positive benefit in reducing cholesterol by at least 10%. Several studies have been performed on garlic oils, and results have been encouraging. However, the dosages used were far above those that are recommended by manufacturers, and the spread of results (that is to say, good and bad) was so wide that further work on these compounds seems unwarranted.

We can now state confidently that allicin is likely to reduce cholesterol by significant amounts in many people and will probably help to reduce the amount of saturated fat absorbed into our bodies. Of course there is always a need for more information and more studies, several of which are underway.

There will always be people who, for one reason or another, will need to take medication to reduce their cholesterol levels. I am not suggesting that allicin is a panacea. Indeed, it is never going to be as effective as some of the prescription medications that are currently available to reduce cholesterol. However, researchers are always keen to compare effects of various alternatives in this kind of treatment, since the patient will have to take medication for the rest of his life. It is therefore important to have a choice. Preferably a number of safe non-drug measures will be tried before a patient is prescribed a specific lipid-lowering drug.

Although there have been controversial discussions concerning the significance of high cholesterol levels for the incidence of arteriosclerosis, several recent studies clearly show that a correlation exists between the concentration of blood lipids and the narrowing of coronary vessels. Some studies, including the large Framingham study, have revealed a significant correlation between serum cholesterol and the risk for heart disease in both men and women. Furthermore, a major 25-year follow-up study in the United States, Europe and Japan has recently shown that increased serum total cholesterol levels are directly associated with increased coronary heart disease across all cultures.

As mentioned earlier, the most important risk factors for developing arteriosclerosis, with its secondary effects such as myocardial infarction, stroke, and occlusive arterial disease, are hyperlipidemia and hypercholesterolemia, in addition to obesity, high blood pressure, diabetes, and nicotine and alcohol abuse.

CIRCULATION
Allicin and blood circulation

Accumulating evidence suggest that allicin may help to improve several parts of your circulation. By making your blood less likely to clot, allicin can reduce blood platelet aggregation. This means that your blood will become slightly thinner and is less likely to form a clot, since the platelets are prevented from sticking together. It has also been reported that allicin will reduce blood thickening. In one study that investigated capillary blood flow in the nail folds of the hand, allicin extracts increased blood flow by 55 per cent in patients who had peripheral arterial occlusive disease (furred up arteries, particularly in the legs).

Sometimes people have circulation defects to almost all of their body. This is called Raynaud's Syndrome. Often, those people affected have to wear gloves even in the warm balmy days of autumn and certainly as the weather begins to cool. Allicin is universally accepted as being able to improve your circulation, and studies show that as soon as you take an allicin capsule, your blood immediately thins and becomes more mobile. It will return to normal within about three hours once the active metabolites constituting allicin have done their work and been excreted.

Treatment regimen

Take 1 to 4 capsules every day, especially during the winter months.

COLD SORES

Medical definition

Inflammation of the skin or mucus membranes caused by the herpes virus and is characterized by a collection of small blisters, especially on the lips. Herpes simplex virus (HSV 1) causes the common cold sore and HSV-2 is responsible for genital herpes. Both types can cause either genital herpes or cold sores depending on the site of the initial infection. HSV blisters are contagious through skin to skin contact and are recurrent in many people.

Most people who are afflicted with recurrent cold sores know exactly when an attack is coming. They will get a tingle on the lips, and if they take action fast enough with allicin liquid, they can prevent that tingle from becoming a full-blown, painful cold sore. Herpes infection arises as a result of some type of toxic insult, which could be stress, infectious illness, food allergies, drug or alcohol abuse, too much sunlight or cold exposure. A significant number of pharmaceutical drugs can also trigger a reaction including, aspirin, motrin, indocin, clinoril and cardizem. Procardia and cortisone are known to increase the invasive nature of herpes virus.

Treatment regimen

Apply just 1 drop of allicin liquid to the sore spot 2 or 3 times a day. This will prevent it from developing into a serious cold sore. At the same time, take 2-4 capsules of allicin powder a day and continue this especially through periods where you might expect to suffer. This protocol should help to prevent the infection from flaring up again.

Testimonials

COLDS AND INFLUENZA
Medical definition

Experts in colds and flu like Professor Ron Eccles, who runs The Common Cold Centre in the UK, will tell you that it is very difficult to determine the difference between a bad cold and a mild flu. Influenza is a highly contagious viral infection that affects the respiratory system. The viruses are transmitted by coughing and sneezing. Symptoms commence after an incubation period of 1-4 days and include headaches, fever, loss of appetite, weakness, sore throat, sneezing, runny nose and general aches and pains. They may continue for about a week, but some people may develop pneumonia, either a primary influenzal viral pneumonia or a secondary bacterial pneumonia. Either of these may be fatal from hemorrhage within the lungs. The main bacterial organisms responsible for a secondary infection include *Streptococcus pneumonia, Heamophilus influenzae* and *Staphylococcus aureus.* All of these bacteria are destroyed by allicin powder capsules.

Classic symptoms of a common cold

Headache, fever, malaise, muscle aches and pains, earache, sinus pain, cough, sneezing, runny nose, sore throat and a blocked nose.

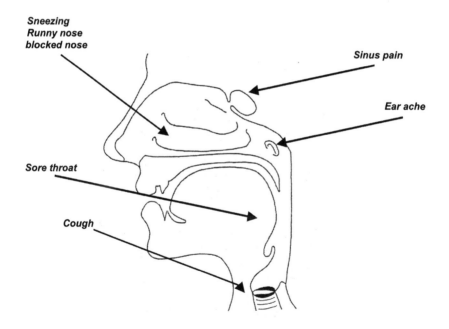

As director of The Garlic Center, I was responsible for conducting the world's first double-blind placebo-controlled study designed to test if allicin powder capsules would be able to prevent and treat the common cold and possibly prevent a recurrent infection.

Our study was published in the peer-reviewed US medical *Journal of Alternatives in Natural Therapy* in 2001. I think that it would be appropriate to record for your interest the study virtually in its entirety.

"The common cold is the world's most widespread viral infection, with most people suffering approximately two to five colds per year. Over 200 different viruses cause infection and cold symptoms; the most common, rhinoviruses, account for 30% to 40% of adult colds. Re-infection is prevalent because of this wide variety of infectious viruses.

"Published literature on the activity of garlic against viral infections is sparse. One report describes that during an influenza epidemic, the former Soviet Union imported more than 500 tons of garlic cloves for acute treatment. Among the viruses sensitive to garlic extracts are the human cytomegalovirus, human rhinovirus type 2, herpes simplex types 1 and 2, and influenza B. Evidence points toward allicin and its condensation product, ajoene, as the main components in garlic responsible for this antiviral activity. Recently, an allicin-containing supplement has demonstrated efficacy against herpes simplex type 1 and molluscum contagiosum infections. A 'cure' for the common cold would substantially reduce the number of work days lost each year as a result of the classic symptoms of infection—tiredness, headaches, a runny nose, sneezing, coughing, watery eyes, and impaired concentration.

"Following recruitment through advertisements in two London daily newspapers, 146 participants were selected. A diary was designed in which each volunteer recorded general well-being for 3 months on a five-point scale.

5 = well, no problems

4 = quite well with occasional sneeze, not disruptive to normal routine

3 = can feel a cold coming on, some minor symptoms

2 = feeling low and beginning to exhibit symptoms

1 = full cold symptoms (headache, sneezing, runny nose, tiredness).

"If a cold occurred, volunteers noted the number and variety of symptoms, the day recovery began, and the day they felt completely better.

"The volunteers were separated into two groups of 73 participants each (matched for sex, age, and garlic consumption). The average age of the participants was 53, and the vast majority were in full time employment. A simple random-number generator assigned volunteers to the active or placebo group, and they were instructed to take one capsule every day with the main meal, according to the manufacturer's recommendation.

"Randomization codes were kept secure at the Garlic Centre and were not broken until all the diaries had been returned. The Garlic Centre contacted volunteers every 2 weeks to ensure that the capsules were being taken correctly and that diary entries were made daily.

"After diaries were returned, the number of colds experienced by volunteers was counted. A cold was defined as a score of 3 that proceeded to 2 or 1, with symptoms. The duration of symptoms was the number of days with a recorded score of 2 or 1, leading to an average recovery time that ended with a score of 4 or 5 taken across all recorded colds. The number of days challenged by the common cold virus was taken as the number of scores of 4 or 3.

"The average symptom length in days and the average number of days challenged by a cold were subjected to calculations of standard deviation, sample variance, and standard error of the difference of the means.

Results

"Four participants withdrew from the study: three from the active group, one from the placebo group. Reasons for withdrawal from active treatment (1 volunteer each) were continued use of another garlic supplement, development of gout, and pruritic rash below the knees, which faded after the allicin supplement was discontinued. The placebo volunteer was advised to discontinue taking the capsules after experiencing severe headaches.

"At the end of the 90-day study, 24 colds were recorded in the active group, 65 in the placebo group. This result is highly significant ($P < 0.001$) in favor of the allicin powder supplement as a cold preventive.

"The placebo group required an average of 5.01 days to recover, compared with 1.58 days in the allicin powder group. This result was statistically significant in favour of the allicin powder group.

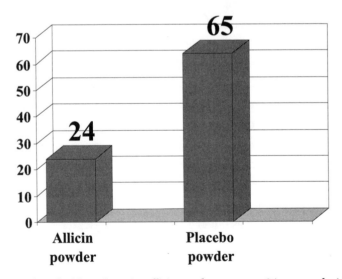

The number of colds in the active allicin powder group was 24 compared with the placebo group who contracted 65 colds. This difference was statistically significant.

"During the study, the 16 volunteers taking the placebo became reinfected (i.e., experienced more than one full-blown cold); only 2 volunteers taking the active supplement had a reinfection.

"Volunteers were also asked to record in their diaries any other concerns during the study, such as comments about the acceptability of taking capsules, side effects, odor, or other reason that might warrant discontinuation of treatment, and to telephone the Garlic Centre if further advice was required.

"Several members of the active group reported increased alertness and feeling generally healthier even though close contacts were falling ill. Some volunteers who took the allicin powder capsules while on holiday noted avoidance of gastric upset and mosquito bites.

"This study is the first to use a double-blind, placebo-controlled design to investigate prevention of viral disease with a garlic supplement. The results overwhelmingly favored the allicin supplement as a preventive measure, demonstrating accelerated relief, reduction in the severity of troublesome symptoms such as sneezing, cough and runny nose, and recovery to full fitness. A reduced likelihood of becoming reinfected with other viral strains indicated general improvement in the immune system with the active supplement.

TREATMENT One capsule per day with food	COLDS	INFECTED DAYS	RECOVERY PERIOD	REPEAT INFECTIONS
ACTIVE (Allicin powder)	24 $p<0.001$	111 $p<0.01$	1.58 $p<0.001$	2 $p<0.05$
PLACEBO (Placebo powder)	65	366	5.01	16

Infected days and recovery period

"Of particular note is that volunteers in the active group took the manufacturer's recommended dose of one capsule per day. Over the past 10 years, other published reports on garlic supplements for numerous applications have often used double or triple the actual dose available in retail outlets.

"The allicin-containing supplement studied may represent a 'cure' for the common cold. The results also suggest that infection and reinfection may be effectively prevented by its daily use throughout the year, with an enormous potential savings to national industry in terms of reduced sick days. This product clearly exhibits excellent antiviral activity and warrants further investigation to determine the nature and method of its viral destruction."

So here is comprehensive, scientifically validated proof that allicin powder capsules can not only prevent the common cold, but treat the symptoms quickly and effectively as well as preventing repeat infections. Surely this alone is enough reason for the vast majority of normal, healthy individuals working in key corporate companies like Microsoft, Dell, Pacific Bell and many others to consider taking allicin.

Testimonials

Mr. CP from Rye in Sussex, England writes, "*Re: My own continuing tests on allicin, I append below my views so far:*

"*As you know I first started using allicin some months ago when I started a heavy cold. I took 4 capsules per day for duration of the cold. The first thing that struck me was that the runny nose cleared up much faster than it would have normally. I continued with 4 a day until the worst of the cold was over after 4 days. I also noted that the usual aftermath of mucus (which usually hangs about because I smoke) was not as severe and cleared more quickly. From that date I reduced the intake to 1 cap per day until I ran out last week! Coincidentally or not, the following day I came down with another heavy cold and unfortunately I did not take any allicin until the end of the week. I immediately took 4 capsules, and have continued until now which is a week from the start. I won't say my cold has cleared, but it is much better. I can breathe clearly and the congestion is beginning to clear (loosen).*

"The other thing which occurs to me, is that I normally feel dreadful when I have a cold for at least 4-5 days, to the point where I do not feel like doing anything. This time I only felt that bad for two days, i.e., Wednesday and Thursday. However, on Friday and through the weekend my energy levels were good despite the fact that I was still heady from cold.

"The other side effect of taking allicin, I have found, is not one of a laxative but more of a regulariser despite the fact that my dietary habits have not changed. This may be coincidence, I do not know.

"There can be little doubt that allicin has beneficial effects. I am a firm believer that treatment from within is the best way to combat ailments, and if the digestive system is working correctly, the body will do the rest. Incidentally, during this time I have only taken the occasional Paracetemol at night to combat headaches."

Mr. CF from Sheerness, Kent, England writes:

"On taking allicin powder capsules for the first time, I encountered several positive experiences, although my feelings on day 3 was of being quite nauseous in the stomach, but after this I started to realise a huge 'clearing' of the airways, almost a slightly runny/mucusey cold.

"As this started to diminish I noticed I could draw large volumes of air through my nose or mouth like I had not done for a good while, what I would call really clear breathing. My wife also commented that I seemed to snore less at this time.

"I continued to take allicin powder capsules on a maintained dose of 1-2 capsules every other day, depending on how I felt. During this

period of approx. 6 months, I never contracted a cold and had good health despite being in the company of others who had colds.

"Then, after stopping the allicin powder capsules for approx. 6 weeks, I contracted a really severe cold. Straight away I started allicin powder capsules again. Within 2 days there was a noticeable improvement. The allicin powder capsules seemed to be reducing the symptoms of the cold; I was certainly recovering quicker than a colleague at work. Then I ran out of allicin powder capsules. This proved to be a disaster, the cold returned with a vengeance and was worse than ever.

"On restarting the allicin powder capsules, the cold symptoms started to lessen, but it proved difficult to shake off, until I doubled the dose. This was large enough to kill it off the second time.

"I can definitely say that there is a relationship between the allicin powder capsules dose/cold symptoms. The point I ran out of the allicin powder capsules and the upturn in the cold symptoms almost seemed symbiotic.

"A cold like this would always go to my chest and result in a sore throat, but this time it hasn't. This is very unusual.

"This product does do something that is difficult to explain and more information is needed on its uses.

"Dosage I took:

"As an everyday supplement: 2 capsules twice a day for 3 days (to start), then 1-2 capsules every other day as maintenance. As a cold cure: 2 x 2 capsules every day (this may have needed to be more)."

Mrs. PMI also from Kent is a sufferer of multiple sclerosis. This means that she has a severely compromised immune system and in previous years has always been highly susceptible to infections. She writes:

Dear Sirs,

Having MS and having no effective immune system, I am certain

that taking allicin powder capsules over the past winter months has helped to protect me from colds and flu. I am pleased to inform you, therefore, that allicin powder capsules with 100% allicin will be a definite part of my future daily intake.
Thank you so much,
Patricia

COUGH and respiratory infections
Preventing coughs

A cough can be the most annoying symptom. It can be unrelenting, and many people may never discover the true cause. We do know that it can have a deep-seated bacterial cause or, in the case of a cold, it is usually a viral infection.

Allicin is known all over the world as a remedy for chest complaints, especially troublesome and persistent coughs, because it has a major antitussive activity. Unlike most, if not all, over-the-counter medicines, allicin powder capsules can destroy both bacterial and viral organisms with consummate ease. This can be achieved in several ways. First, gargle with allicin liquid that has been added to a little milk or water. Take 10 drops of allicin liquid and add this to a small cupful of warm milk. Gargle for a few minutes. Do this every night for a few days. Then, before retiring to bed, take 6 allicin powder capsules and continue this until the cough begins to break up. Reduce the dose to 4 and then to 2 after a further week.

CRYPTOSPORIDIUM
Medical definition

This is a parasitic infection caused by a protozoan that comes from infected human and animal excrement commonly found in soil and fresh water. In recent years this has become a much more widespread problem.

Recent outbreaks include the now famous Milwaukee incident of 1993. It is reported that 400,000 people developed the infection from drinking contaminated water. There were dozens of fatalities. Recent reports in Great Britain and Canada also traced the infection to contaminated water supplies requiring large numbers of people to boil all water for domestic use for several months. With no effective drug medications or water sterilants available, this particular parasite will continue to cause panic and attract world-wide publicity for some time to come.

The AIDS Research Alliance in California has been testing the effectiveness of allicin in combating cryptosporidosis. The parasite is thought to burrow into the intestinal wall and may invade both red blood cells and liver cells. It protects itself from destruction by converting itself into a cyst. The tests involved patients taking liquid allicin mixed with distilled water twice daily. Patients suffered from less diarrhea and had a stable or increasing body weight. For several patients, repeated testing showed negative results for cryptosporidium parasites. Larger trials are planned.

Treatment regimen

Treatment will need to be aggressive and prolonged to have a chance of destroying this parasite. A large dose, 10 a day, of allicin powder capsules should be taken all at once or spread throughout the day. It would also be sensible to take 10 drops of allicin liquid in fruit juice twice a day for the entire treatment period. Results will depend on each individuals response, but don't be afraid to persevere as the allicin can only do you good.

DANDRUFF

Medical definition

Visible scaling from the surface of the scalp is extremely common and is evident in at least 50% of the population. Dandruff is caused by the yeast, Pityrosporum ovale, *and is often the precursor of seborrhoeic eczema of the scalp. This is usually accompanied by a degree of inflammation and greasy scaling.*

Most people don't realize that dandruff is caused by a fungal infection, and most of the proprietary shampoos and conditioners do not contain any antifungal agents at all. Consequently, very little impact is made on a scalp that is infected, yet Americans spend millions of dollars each year on the latest cosmetic products that, with expensive marketing campaigns, guarantee success—for the manufacturers!

Allicin liquid can be mixed with any shampoo or conditioner and, with just a few applications, will get rid of dandruff very easily. It is necessary to adopt what I call the "heal from within and heal from without" principle. This means that you must start taking allicin powder capsules at the same time, since we are trying to get rid of an infection and then prevent it from coming back. At the same time, men will notice that they will lose less hair when adding allicin liquid into any ordinary shampoo. This is because the allicin gets absorbed into the scalp and penetrates the hair follicles, improving the blood supply and lessening the opportunities for hair loss. Try it and see for yourself!

Treatment regimen

Add 8 drops of allicin liquid to a normal measure of shampoo and massage as usual in the last wash. You can then use a conditioner if necessary. Repeat this every time you wash your hair for about 1 month. At the same time start taking just 1 capsule of allicin powder every day and continue this for preventing the infection from returning.

DIABETES

A personal testimonial

Since diabetics are three times more likely to suffer from cardiovascular disease than a normal individual, are less able to fight off infections and will heal much more slowly than non-diabetics, allicin powder capsules can offer a cascade of benefits.

" I have not had ANY colds despite having 2 young children at school! I can attribute this to allicin. "

As the author of this book, I have a unique experience with the production and application of allicin. I am also a diabetic of some 32 years standing, so anything I can do to reduce the risks detailed above has to be good for me. Consequently, I take allicin capsules every day to help keep my blood pressure, cholesterol and circulation fit and healthy. Anyone who knows me will tell you that before the advent of allicin powder capsules, I used to take a popular garlic powder supplement. Every year around October I would get a real stinker of a cold. This would usually last at least 10 days, since my immune system doesn't function as well as the immune system of a non-diabetic, and my blood sugar levels would go haywire. Since starting allicin powder capsules several years ago, I have not had ANY colds despite now having 2 young children at school! I can only attribute this to allicin.

Diabetics, myself included, also tend to heal very slowly. I still have a scar from a minor burn I sustained when I was a teenager, and every time I cut myself, it seems to take ages to heal properly. Recently, however, I have started putting allicin liquid onto plasters or bandages used to dress small cuts and grazes. A short time ago I got a nasty wood splinter in my thumbnail. I managed to remove it, but immediately it started to swell up a little and became very painful. I immediately added just 3 drops of allicin liquid to a band-aid and dressed the wound. Literally within a few hours, the pain and swelling had begun to reduce and I changed the dressing the next day. Within 3-4 days, the wound had healed, the swelling was gone and it was not painful at all. Several days later, having stopped the treatment, my skin began to flake and peel away, leaving a perfectly healed thumb. Allicin really is great stuff for diabetics!

DIAPER RASH

Medical definition

A red skin rash, within the diaper area, is usually caused by chemical irritation (ammoniacal dermatitis) or infection with Candida. Ammoniacal dermatitis is caused by skin contact with a soiled diaper. The stool bacteria react with urine to form the irritant ammonia.

Allicin creme has the consistency and quality to be used as a diaper rash treatment. It contains 125ppm allicin (parts per million), and it is well documented that allicin can kill fungal infections at a concentration as low as 1.7ppm!

Treatment regimen

Each morning apply a thin covering of allicin creme all over the diapered area. If possible, do not allow your baby to sit in a soiled diaper for very long before changing. Apply the creme every time you change your baby.

DIARRHEA

Medical definition

Frequent bowel evacuation or the passage of abnormally soft or liquid feces, often caused by intestinal infection, especially by Escherichia coli. *Severe or prolonged diarrhea may lead to extreme loss of fluids, salt and nutrients.*

Treatment regimen

Diarrhea is easily combated with allicin powder capsules. All you need to do is take a large dose—once—and this will get rid of an upset stomach. Take 6 allicin capsules in one dose. In severe case, this may have to be repeated six hours later.

I can personally guarantee that this works. As a person who sometimes gets a stomach upset leading to terrible stomach pains followed by the classic "explosion," I have always relied on pharmaceutical preparations, which certainly do work, but I much prefer to use allicin since it is safe, natural and very effective!

DELAYED AGING

There has been an impressive gain in individual life expectancy with parallel increases in age-related chronic diseases of the cardiovascular, brain and immune systems. These can cause loss of autonomy, dependence and high social costs for individuals and society. It is now accepted that aging and age-related diseases are in part caused by free radical reactions.

The arrest of aging and stimulation of rejuvenation of the human body is also being sought. Over the last 20 years, the use of herbs and natural products has gained popularity, backed by epidemiological evidence. One such herb is garlic, which has been used throughout the history of civilization for treating a wide variety of ailments associated with aging.

The role of garlic in preventing age-related diseases has been investigated extensively over the last 10-15 years. Garlic has strong antioxidant properties and it has been suggested that garlic can combat cardiovascular disease, inhibit platelet aggregation and thrombus formation; fight cancer, diseases associated with cerebral aging, arthritis, cataract formation; rejuvenate skin; and improve blood circulation and energy levels. This review provides an insight into garlic's antioxidant properties and presents evidence that it may either prevent or delay chronic diseases associated with aging.

The beneficial effects claimed for the use of garlic as a nutritional supplement include detoxification, antioxidation, antifungal activity, antibacterial activity, tumour suppression and, possibly, anti-aging and rejuvenating effects. We have used the Hayflick system of cellular aging in culture in order to test garlic for its anti-aging effects on long-term growth characteristics, morphology and macromolecular synthesis of human skin fibroblasts. Results show that an addition of garlic extract into the normal cell culture medium can support serial subculturing for more than 55 population doublings in 475 days, and that this treatment has some youth-preserving, anti-aging and beneficial effects on human fibroblasts in terms of maximum proliferative capacity and morphological characteristics. In comparison, similar or lesser doses of garlic extracts are growth inhibitory for cancerous cells that could not be grown over longer periods in the presence of garlic. To our knowledge, this is the first report of the effects of garlic on the long-term growth characteristics and macromolecular synthesis of normal human skin cells, the results of which have applications for both anti-aging and anti-cancer research.

We suggest the regular intake of allicin powder capsules at the recommended daily dose of between 180mg and 560mg per day.

EAR INFECTIONS

For a young child, an ear infection is difficult to live with. It can be impossible for your child to communicate the pain and discomfort he or she is suffering. Naturally, a caring parent wants to get a quick resolution. A trip to the doctor will result immediately in a prescription for an antibiotic drug which will probably work. But a cursory look at the medical databases shows that when children are aggressively treated with antibiotics, they become 300% more likely to develop recurrent infections when compared to those who have no treatment at all. Since children are still developing an effective immune system, over use of antibiotics can easily result in a fungal infection.

Treatment regimen

Any condition that has a microbial cause can be treated with allicin. For a child under 7 years old, give 2 capsules a day, split open, and place the powder in their food. You can also drizzle the liquid into the ear just 1 drop at a time for a period of up to 1 week.

EYE INFECTIONS

Testimonial

"First of all, thank you for introducing us to allicin capsules. After hearing so many positive things about it, we were all willing to give it a try.

"I think they too have been very surprised by the results."

"In July I had a very bad eye infection. I went to the doctor and was prescribed an eye ointment called "Brolene." I had to apply this morning and evening, and was told by the doctor if there was no improvement, to go back to surgery. After the first day of applying Brolene, the next morning my eyes had a sticky residue which I had to battle with salty water to separate the eye lashes. I carried on, but after a couple of days, my eyes were still red and sore.

"I then went back to the doctor as there was no improvement at all. I was then prescribed an antibiotic eye cream, which again I had to apply two drops morning and evening. If no better, I was to go back to my doctor.

"This continued with two different creams and still no improvement, I persevered for a further two days, but was beginning, by this time, to get really fed up as my eyes were no better at all.

"I then tried the allicin capsules, taking two per day for two days. On the first day the itchiness had stopped and the redness became less. Then on the second day my eyes were completely clear.

"I was so impressed that I have told friends and work colleagues about your product. As for myself, after taking allicin for two days, the difference was unbelievable, especially after going to the doctor and using their prescriptions to no avail.

"As soon as friends mention they've got a pain or a sniffle they are all quite keen to try allicin, and I think they, too, have been very surprised by the results. Thank you again.
Yours sincerely,
Mrs. C Francis, Sussex, England

EBOLA AND DENGUE FEVER

Both of these serious diseases are caused by a virus known as arbovirus, related to hemorraghic fever. These infections are rare in the United States, but with people traveling into the country from all over the world, it is easy to bring not only your luggage with you, but an infectious virus as well.

The syndrome of "viral hemorrhagic fever" in man caused by certain viruses, such as Ebola, Lassa, Dengue, and Crimean-Congo hemorrhagic fever viruses, is often associated with a shock syndrome of undetermined cause. The vascular system, particularly the vascular endothelium, seems to be directly and indirectly targeted by all these viruses. Infections with these filoviruses show lethality up to 89%, and in severe cases lead to a shock syndrome associated with hypotension, coagulation disorders and an imbalance of fluid distribution between the intravascular and extravascular tissue space. The primary target cells for filoviruses are mononuclear phagocytotic cells, which are activated upon infection and release certain cytokines and chemokines. These mediators indirectly target the endothelium and are thought to play a key role in the pathogenesis of filoviral hemorrhagic fever. In addition, direct infection and subsequent destruction of endothelial cells might contribute to the pathogenesis. Filoviruses, particularly Ebola virus, encode nonstructural glycoproteins, which are released from infected host cells.

So once again, infection is the root cause. Allicin, is an excellent anti-viral that can boost the immune system, while at the same time not disturb your healthy bacterial flora, and may be able to help significantly in protecting you from a viral challenge.

The last case of a serious outbreak of dengue fever in the United States was in the southwestern United States with over 700,000 people infected just in Texas. Only recently in 2002, West Nile Virus spread across many US states, so now is the time to get protection by adding a daily dose of allicin capsules for each member of the family.

ECZEMA
Medical definition
This is a common itchy skin disease characterized by reddening and vesicle formation which may lead to weeping and crusting. Atopic eczema affects up to 20% of the population and is associated with hay fever and asthma. It can affect young children, in particular, and the disease may last for several years leading on into adulthood.

Most people who suffer from eczema will have their own routine that at least keeps the disease at bay. It could involve a number of pharmaceutical agents, including steroids plus emollients, and a wide variety of herbal remedies are also routinely used. However, most sufferers will also report that these treatments work for a short period of time and then, for some reason, cease to be effective and the formulations have to be changed.

One of the major reasons for this tolerance developing to a plethora of agents used to help treat eczema is that NONE of them (including many pharmaceutical drugs) can kill the bacterium that is found in 95% of simple cases of eczema—a beast called *Staphylococcus aureus*.

The table below shows just how often this bug is found all over the skin surface of eczema sufferers. This bacterium is clever and will selectively seek out a route into the human body (see MRSA section later), so an eczema patient is the ideal vehicle for *Staphylococcus aureus* to replicate and infect. Its prescence on the skin will cause a secondary infection, which leads to a worsening of clinical symptoms and will prevent the absorption of hydrocortisone as well.

Percentage prevelance of Staphylococcus aureus infection	Normal individuals	Eczema sufferers
NOSE	34	59
CHEEK	7	63
CHEST	3	48
FOREARM	2	63
SCAPULA	2	46

So it stands to reason that you must use an agent that can kill *Staphyloccocus aureus* and allow the underlying disease to heal. Allicin can do this easily. So far over 80 strains of this infectious multi-drug-resistant bacteria have been tested against allicin liquid powder and creme formulations and have all been blown away!

Treatment regimen

Begin by starting a high-dose course of allicin powder capsules. Take up to 6 a day. At the same time take a few drops of allicin liquid or creme and apply sparingly to your eczema plaques. Do this twice a day for a month or until you begin to see improvement. Continue to take the capsules on a daily basis at a reduced dose of 1-2 capsules per day.

FUNGAL NAIL DISEASE
Medical definition

This is incredibly common in the Western World and, in particular, the United States, where many millions of people suffer in silence. Caused by Dermatophytes and Candida albicans, the fungus invades the toe or fingernails feeding off the rich supply of keratin found deep in the nail beds.

A number of factors will increase the liklehood of developing nail fungus. These include poor hygiene, a sugary diet, application of artificial nails and nail polish. Sadly, yeast infections like this can often start from within our body, so it is important to use an agent like allicin that can heal from within as well as treat the condition from without (that is topically). You will have seen the picture of toenail fungus inside the front cover of this book, and if you haven't already followed the footsteps to the inside back cover, please do so now! Amazing, wasn't it?

That patient would have almost certainly lost his big toenail without treatment. It was beginning to split and crack. Within a very short period of time, the nail would have started to break away, and he may never have grown another one. Fortunately, we encouraged him to use allicin liquid and creme products, and you have seen the results. After just a few weeks, the fungus was destroyed and his nail was clean and healthy.

Treatment regimen

Simply apply a small dab of allicin creme or liquid to each infected nail. If you have a fungus on your fingernails, add just 1 drop of allicin liquid to each nail twice daily. To prevent a recurrent infection, take allicin capsules regularly (2 per day). One other interesting benefit from applying the liquid to fingernails is that it makes them much stronger and far less likely to crack or split. You can just apply one drop per nail before you add your colour, and within a few weeks, you will notice a significant difference to the quality of your nails.

GINGIVITIS
Medical definition

Inflammation of the gums caused by plaque on the surfaces of the teeth at their necks. The gums are swollen and bleed easily. This can lead to periodontal disease, but is reversible with good oral hygiene.

The composition of the plaque which causes gingivitis includes a number of bacterial species. Gums are growing tissue that require a consistent supply of nutrients for continued good health. Once the gums begin to degenerate, a number of pockets can develop where food particles can accumulate and act as a magnet for further bacterial overgrowth. This leads to the release of a wide range of toxins that continue the cycle of decay. Allicin powder can be easily placed on a number of foodstuffs to be chewed in the mouth. This will help to remove the various bacterial strains that infect our oral cavities.

Treatment regimen

Break open 2 allicin powder capsules per day and place the powder over your favorite food product and chew in your mouth. This will help to cleanse your mouth of bacteria.

HAY FEVER

Medical definition

Hay fever is an allergic reaction to pollen, trees, grasses and other plants, characterized by inflammation of the membrane lining the nose and sometimes the conjunctiva.

There are approximately 12 million sufferers of hay fever in the UK and over 75 million in the USA. Symptoms vary from mild discomfort to those that are so severe that the sufferer cannot even go outdoors. One of the most recent peer-reviewed studies that I have performed investigated hay fever prevention and treatment with allicin powder capsules. The following is a summary taken from the research paper published in *The British Journal of Clinical Phytomedicine* in 2002.

An allergic reaction is caused when the immune system mistakenly identifies a normally harmless substance as a threat. The reason why some people are allergic to substances such as pollen is unknown, but the cause may be genetic.

The body's allergic response is triggered by the immune system reacting with mast cells that are found in or near a variety of organs and tissues, including the nose, lungs, skin, eyes and blood vessels. These mast cells contain high concentrations of histamine, which is released when stimulated by the body's immune defences.

Histamine, when released in the body, induces many responses. These responses are known as hay fever when the cause is pollen released by plants. Symptoms of hay fever include:

- a congested and itchy nose
- a constantly running nose
- the eyes become very itchy and watery
- the eyelids become swollen and itchy
- breathing can become difficult
- there may be loss of taste and hearing
- dry cough
- headache

The symptoms vary in severity from person to person and in response to high or low pollen counts, which vary by the day and weather conditions.

Antihistamines are used to prevent the release of histmanine from mast cells or to diminish the effect after the histamine has been released.

Oral antihistamines are probably the most convenient treatment for most people. There are two main types.

The older types cause drowsiness because they cross the blood-brain barrier. Examples of this type include Piriton, Phenergan, and Haymine. The newer types or non-sedating antihistamines are better tolerated and include Clarityn, Benadryl, Singulair and Zyrtek.

Antihistamines differ in their duration of action and in side effects. Generally, the newer non-sedating products are longer acting and have fewer side effects than the older drugs, and all products noted above are available for sale without prescripton from pharmacies.

There are also antihistamines available only on prescription such as

Telfast, Neoclarityn (non-sedating) and Vallergan and Atarax, which are sedating antihistamines.

Eye drops and nasal sprays are also available. These are preferred by some patients because they perceive that these products are more efficacious because of the direct application. However, for effective treatment the products have to be used frequently. Examples of eye drops (the most widely-used drug is sodium cromoglycate) include Opticrom and Optrex, which contain sodium cromoglycate and work by preventing release of histamine. Users must be reminded not to use this type of product when wearing contact lenses. Patients suffering from conditions such as glaucoma should also avoid this type of product.

Nasal sprays, such as beclomethasone, are also available for sale through pharmacies and work by reducing inflammation and mucous production. They should not be used in cases of nasal infection, and these products are not licensed for sale over the counter for patients under 18 years old.

Historically, many types of garlic preparation, varying from fresh crushed raw garlic to heavily-processed powder products have been used to treat diseases of respiratory origin including asthma, bronchitis, allergies and inflammation. Interestingly, it has been shown that garlic extracts are capable of inhibiting histamine release from basophils and mast cells as well as inhibiting lipoxygenase in neutrophils. For many years, garlic has been used extensively in Third World Countries as a simple, modestly effective trestment for a wide range of respiratory disease.

The many garlic supplements marketed in the United Kingdom, United States and Europe vary widely by type and definition of active constituents. Increasing evidence has shown that certain forms of supplement may have significant beneficial properties, provided that the universally recognized active constituent (allicin) is made available to the body.

A survey was designed to determine whether stabilized allicin powder capsules could prevent the classic ay fever attack from occurring among volunteers who have suffered for some years.

Following recruitment through a local radio station, 29 volunteers were enrolled in the late Spring of 2001. A diary was designed in which each volunteer recorded general well-being for the study period of 35 days.

A five-point scale was used:

5 = Well, no problems
4 = Quite well with occasional sneeze
3 = Can feel an attack coming on, some minor symptoms
2 = Feeling low and definitely suffering
1 = Full hay fever attack with symptoms listed

Volunteers were instructed to record the number and variety of symptoms, the day recovery began, and the day they felt completely better. They were asked to take 2 capsules of allicin powder each day with food in accordance with the manufacturer's recommendations.

Volunteers were also told that if a full hay fever attack occurred, they could revert to drug treatment if necessary. This was recorded in the diary.

The pollen count was monitored and recorded every day throughout the study period using both local and national information sources.

- The overall AVERAGE SCORE was 3.95, indicating that allicin powder capsules were able to control hay fever very well.
- Over 80% of volunteers reported a significant reduction in the number of challenges throughout the study period.
- Only 2 volunteers needed to resort to drug treatment for an attack.
- Most volunteers were impressed with the treatment and claimed that their hay fever was "much better," controlled with allicin powder capsules.

- Volunteers reported far fewer symptoms than they expected, with big reductions in "sore eyes," "runny nose," "itching at the back of the throat," "sneezing" and "tiredness."
- Everyone found allicin capsules easy to take and did not report any side effects. There were no reports of odor while taking this product.

Generally, the volunteers reported that allicin powder capsules were easy to take and rather effective. Although the treatment did not work for everyone and some comments indicated that the "season" was finishing, most volunteers were extremely positive and included observations that previous drug treatment had never really removed all symptoms, whereas allicin powder casules did. People were more able to go about their normal daily routine without interruption from troublesome symptoms. One gentleman reported being able to play golf 3 times a week without any problems—apart from the golf! Another young lady was able to sit out on fresh mown lawn for the first time since her hay fever symptoms developed in her teens. Other unsolicited comments included volunteers being able to mix and socialise without worrying about running noses and streaming eyes.

Our pilot investigation clearly shows that allicin-based supplements have an ability to prevent allergic reaction to pollen and may offer a safe and natural alternative to pharmaceutical preparations. The treatment should be started as early as possible and continued throughout the season. For many people, this represents a real chance to reduce the number of compromises that hay fever sufferers have to make each year.

Treatment regimen

With the above study it is clear that a daily dose of just 2 allicin capsules per day can dramatically reduce the number of hay fever attacks that sufferers are likely to experience.

Testimonial

Here are some extracts from a diary kindly forwarded to me by Zoe M, a young lady who contracted hay fever at a young age and who has experienced just about every pharmaceutical drug manufactured to treat her symptoms—mostly to no avail. We asked her to try allicin capsules during the spring when her hay fever is usually at its worst. I have inserted the local pollen count for her area in Sussex, England, for each day that she made an entry into her diary.

Allicin capsule diary by hayfever sufferer, Zoe M

Monday 15 May

Very warm day today and very muggy. Took my first dose (2 capsules). Felt a little less stuffed up by the evening but still suffering quite badly from a heavy pollen count over the weekend. [Pollen count HIGH]

Tuesday 16 May

It has been a little cooler today and have felt the benefits. Continued with the 2 capsules dosage, I cannot tell whether me feeling better is down to the capsules or the weather clearing a little. My nose is clearer and sore throat has gone completely. [Pollen count HIGH]

Wednesday 17 May

Feel completely clear today. Sore throat has not come back and nose is clear. Still taking the 2 capsules. [Pollen count MEDIUM]

Thursday 18 May

Didn't even sneeze once today—did blow my nose though! Feeling fine, actually a little bit lively. 2 capsules again today. [Pollen count MEDIUM]

Friday 19 May

Feeling absolutely fine, no problems. [Pollen count HIGH]

Saturday 20 May

It has been a little warmer today—still no blocked nose or streaming eyes, which are my usual tell-tale signs. [Pollen count HIGH]

Sunday 21 May
No problems today. [Pollen count LOW]
Monday 22 May
They cut the grass outside our flats today, which usually sets me off, but no problems at all. It smells quite nice and it is nice to be able to smell it at all!
Still taking the recommended dosage 2 capsules. [Pollen count MEDIUM]
Tuesday 23 May
Fine, no problems. [Pollen count HIGH]
Wednesday 24 May
Fine, no problems. [Pollen count MEDIUM]
Thursday 25 May
Fine, no problems. [Pollen count MEDIUM]
Friday 26 May
Very bunged up this morning—but blew nose just once and ok – this didn't continue throughout the day as normal. [Pollen count VERY HIGH]
Saturday 27 May
Feel fine today. [Pollen count HIGH]

This really is quite amazing. For the first time ever I have been able to go about my normal routine without sneezing and constantly feeling blocked up. This allicin product is definitely the best thing I have ever used for treating my hay fever.
Thanks ever so much,
Zoe

HEAD LICE

Control of infections with head lice has traditionally been performed using conventional insecticides. Historically, these materials have been appropriate for killing the insects and their eggs, but recently problems have arisen in several parts of the world due to the selection of strains of lice that have developed resistance to one or more insecticides. Consumers have become disillusioned by these "conventional" agents, which are also highly inflammable and rather toxic to the human body, especially our children. With many existing products making claims that can no longer be justified, the desire to find alternative therapy has prompted many consumers to experiment and resort to untested methods. Also, a number of formulators have decided to market products that are neither adequately tested for safety or efficacy, nor are they licensed products for use in this application. Some materials used in this application are potentially toxic and, because many of the formulations are inappropriate, may encourage the development of resistance to some of the potentially available alternative active substances.

The purpose of the tests reproduced below was to establish the efficacy of Allisure Allicin Liquid against adult head lice with an overnight test followed by a second test the next day on the remaining live lice.

Human lice, *Pediculus humanus*, were obtained from the culture colony maintained by Insect R&D Limited. Adult female and male lice, in approximately equal numbers, were used for pediculicidal tests. The lice were fed on the morning of the test and allowed a minimum of 4 hours to recover, during which time they were able to excrete excess water imbibed with their blood meal. Lice were counted into batches of twenty and were provided with squares of open-meshed nylon gauze (tulle), as a substrate upon which to stand, and each batch was allocated to a marked 30 millimetre plastic petri dish.

Pediculicidal tests

For the test procedure, an aliquot of approximately 5-10 millilitres of allicin liquid was poured into the base of a clean 30 millimetre plastic petri dish. The gauze bearing the lice was immersed in the fluid for 10 seconds, during which time the gauze was turned at least twice to ensure removal of air bubbles. After removal from the fluid, the gauze and insects were lightly blotted to remove excess fluid and returned to their marked petri dish. The same procedure was repeated for the other replicate gauze squares in that batch.

Gauze squares bearing the lice were incubated under normal maintenance conditions (30° ± 2° Celsius and 50% ± 15% relative humidity) overnight. At the end of the exposure period, the insects and gauze were washed using a bland toiletry shampoo or frequent wash shampoo. The lice were then fed a blood meal and left for 4 hours to recover before being treated once again as above. The results were read at 24 hours and 48 hours.

The control batches for this test were treated with 60% IPA (Propan-2-ol) as above.

Activity against lice

The tests with the allicin formulation show that with an overnight exposure it had effect on the lice with an overall mortality of 57.8% compared to that of the controls at 11.0%. However, after a blood meal and a second treatment, the results show 98.4% mortality, with the controls having 28.6%

Test	Dead	Alive	Morbid	Mortality
Day 1				
A1	5	11	7	52.2 %
A2	9	7	5	66.7 %
A3	7	9	4	55.0 %
Total	21	27	16	57.8 %
C1	2	18	0	11.0 %
Day 2				
A1	22	1	1	95.8 %
A2	19	0	2	100 %
A3	15	0	5	100 %
Total	56	1	8	98.4 %
C1	4	14	0	28.6 %

Results of tests against adult lice with allicin liquid

These initial tests were very good. Clearly, allicin can be safely used to treat and probably prevent a lice infestation in your children!

Treatment regimen

We have used this regimen at home on both our daughters with great success. Take a normal scoop of your favorite shampoo and add 20 drops of allicin liquid. Mix thoroughly and then shampoo the hair as normal. Like a conditioner, leave the shampoo on for a couple of minutes and then wash off and repeat again. One bottle of allicin liquid will give you at least 11 treatments. This procedure should be repeated every day for a week. This will ensure that the eggs and nits are removed. At the same time, you must use all the normal measures recommended by public health experts. So please ensure that you treat everyone in the family (including Dad), and that you thoroughly comb out any shells, eggs or dead lice that may still be stuck to the hair. At the end of the week, your child's hair should be clean and nit free, but it is probably worthwhile using this technique once or twice the following week to prevent a reinfestation, since you can bet that somebody at school won't be as thorough as you!

HEAVY METAL CONTAMINATION
Allicin detoxifies heavy metals

We have known about this feature of allicin's medicinal activities for a long time. There are many reports of water-based extracts of garlic being used as a cleanser to clear poisonous metals from the blood. Recent work has centered on proving that allicin can reduce the absorption of lead by farm animals. As our population grows, it becomes more difficult to find enough land to give to farmers and their livestock. We continue to pollute our atmosphere at an alarming rate. Thus it comes as a pleasant surprise to learn that allicin liquid is being used to ensure that chickens and other livestock do not absorb dangerous quantities of toxic metals like lead from the atmosphere. It has even been calculated that the amount of lead that WE now absorb from the atmosphere has increased a thousandfold over the last century! Many people are now also worried about mercury poisioning from tooth fillings, and this is another metal that can be removed quite efficiently from our bodies using a detox formula that contains allicin.

HEPATITIS
Medical definition

This is inflammation of the liver and can be caused by viruses, toxic substances or immunological abnormalities. There are many different types, some transmitted sexually and others through an exchange of body fluids from an infected person.

Hepatitis is very difficult to treat. Every year around 400,000 Americans develop a Hepatitis B or C infection. Many of the viruses that can cause hepatitis are from the herpetic family and will also include Epstein-Barr-type viral infections. We already know that allicin has the capability to destroy and prevent these organisms from flare up in the human body. So allicin formulations will have some benefit, but the complexity and very nature of hepatitis make it difficult to show results. However, the natural boost to the immune system that allicin can give will have some beneficial effect.

Treatment regimen

Take a large dose of allicin capsules—up to 10 per day over a prolonged period. It may be worthwhile diluting the liquid by half and taking it internally every day. A half a fluid ounce twice daily is recommended.

IMMUNE SYSTEM

The human immune system operates as a complex mixture of biochemical and cellular interactions. A wide range of organs and cells provide the basic components for the system. These are the lymphatic vessels and organs (lymph nodes, thymus, spleen, and tonsils), white blood cells such as lymphocytes and monocytes and specialized cells residing in various tissues responsible for phagocytosis (macrophages). Phagocytosis occurs when macrophages engulf and eat invading microorganisms or cancer cells.

There are two major types of immune response, the relatively instant innate response and the slower adaptive response.

The innate responses include:

- physical barriers such as skin
- mechanical responses such as mucus production, (to trap and remove)
- chemicals such as fatty acids on the skin, acid in the stomach and complement in the blood to assist phagocytosis
- macrophages (phagocytic cells)
- natural killer cells or killer T cells

Natural killer cells produce a non-specific response that acts directly against viruses and cancer cells. Natural killer cells attack any body cells with a changed surface. When viruses invade your cells, they can change the outer surface of the cell and tumor cells often have changes in their outer surface proteins. Natural killer cells are therefore very important to rapid protection and daily maintenance of your body.

The adaptive responses relate mainly to the production of specific antibodies against a "non-self" stimulus. Active immunity against a microbe you have not met before can take two to three weeks to develop. This is why the body requires the two lines of defense, the rapid and the slower responses. Immune cells circulate throughout the body to kill invading bacteria, yeasts, virus, fungi or cancer cells. The major cell types involved are lymphocytes, T (thymus) cells (killer cells and helper cells), and B (bone marrow) cells. B cells give rise to antibody-producing plasma cells. T helper cells then help B cells react specifically with antigens (non-self stimulators, e.g., bacteria or viruses).

There are also non-cellular "chemical" components of the immune system which complement proteins that kill targeted invading cells and regulate inflammatory responses and cytokines, such as the interleukins and interferons. Cytokines are very important chemicals that act as messengers between the cells that secrete them and their cellular targets. They are like the body's "cruise missile" targeting system, only more accurate.

It is clear that the immune system, the way the body defends itself against disease, is complex and multi-faceted. We still do not know all of its secrets. However, there are aspects of the immune system that can be examined in a laboratory setting.

In the laboratory, one can examine the ability of these agents to stimulate the immune system cells (natural killer cells and macrophages) mentioned above, and we can also examine the ability of the agent to inhibit and kill the invading micro-organism or tumor cells. Both of these tests would give an indication of how the agent may stimulate the immune system and assist the immune system in protecting against invasion. These tests help to decide whether or not new agents have the POTENTIAL to act as immunomodulators. The evidence gained from these must be followed by evidence provided from properly controlled clinical trials.

Allicin powder capsules

As we have established, allicin is the principle active agent in fresh aqueous garlic (*Allium sativum*) extracts. Sanskrit (a very ancient Indian language) records document the use of garlic as a medicine some 5000 years ago. The Egyptian *Codex Eber Papyrus* (B.C. 1550) mentions garlic as an effective remedy for a wide variety of ailments. We have also confirmed that allicin is a natural antibiotic and in the past has been variously used to

1) Protect the body from infection
2) Detoxify the body
3) Strengthen blood vessels and
4) Lower blood pressure

A mixture of garlic and vinegar known as the "four thieves" was credited with protecting the citizens of Marseilles from catching the plague in 1722. Throughout the centuries in India, France, Germany, Denmark and Switzerland, garlic extracts have been used to treat bronchitis, colds, hay fever, and asthma.

The biological activity of allicin is thought to be related to a combination of factors:

1) Its activity as an antioxidant
2) Its ability to attack the sulphur (SH) groups in enzymes and proteins and modify their activity and
3) Its ability to rapidly penetrate into cells through the cell membranes

Allicin has a number of beneficial properties which could act together to enhance the body's response to disease. Published laboratory studies have found that allicin:

- Enhances the activity of phagocytic cells
- Enhances the activity of natural killer cells
- Inhibits the growth of pathogenic micro-organisms and
- Inhibits the growth of certain cancer cell

One of the main problems with laboratory studies has been the purity of the extracts used. Only recently has a purified, natural, stable extract of allicin become available for testing. Recent studies in London have confirmed the antibacterial activity of this stabilized allicin extract against a number of different bacteria, including multiple antibiotic-resistant *Staphylococcus aureus* (MRSA). Further clinical trials with this substance are underway.

Clinical Trials

In the USA, trials in AIDS patients have demonstrated enhancement of natural killer cell activity using garlic extracts, and Chinese studies with viral infections in bone marrow transplant patients have demonstrated a "potent antiviral activity." Human population studies have shown that regular intake reduces the risk of esophageal, stomach and colon cancer. This was thought to be due to the antioxidant effect of allicin in reducing the formation of carcinogenic compounds in the gastrointestinal tract. A small survey using allicin powder (Allisure) has reported that allicin can reduce the occurrence of colds and flu and the length of the symptoms.

Allicin has the potential to assist the immune system in a number of different ways, stimulating immune cells, killing pathogens and detoxifying carcinogens. Although the compound can be obtained directly from fresh garlic bulbs, one would have to regularly eat large amounts of cooked garlic to obtain any beneficial effect and few of us can eat large amounts of raw garlic. This leaves us with liquids and powders. Given the importance of the agent, any garlic liquids or powders should give an indication of the amount of allicin available from the product, but many do not.

In January 2000, *Toronto Star* reporter, Leslie Papp, examined a number of "herbal cures" including garlic. The imminent opening of Canada's new Office of Natural Health Products prompted this investigation. Of the three herbal products tested, they found "None of the three brands of garlic supplements met their claims of how much allicin they could produce. Yet allicin is the ingredient used to measure the potency of the product."

Taking too much allicin (or garlic) may hinder blood clotting. Allicin should not be taken by people already on anticoagulants or those about to undergo surgery *without* previously informing the health care physician in charge. It may also cause reactions in people allergic to garlic, although this has only been reported once to my knowledge!

IMPETIGO
Medical definition
Impetigo is a superficial bacterial infection of the skin caused by Stapylococcus aureus *infection. It mainly affects young children and is highly infectious, causing a yellow-brown crusting on the skin.*

For a young child, this can be a particularly distressing condition, since all their friends have to be warned "do not touch" because it is so infectious. Once again the bacterial specie involved is *Staphylococcus*, which is highly sensitive to allicin treatment.

Treatment regimen
For children under the age of 5, it is best to remove the powder from the capsule and spread the allicin over the child's favorite food or dissolve it in a juice drink. For older children, gently apply 2 drops of

allicin liquid every 4 hours and dose 4 allicin capsules per day until the outbreak subsides. If your child has contact with any friends or family members, everyone should take 1-2 capsules a day to prevent the infection from being passed on to others.

Testimonial

Mum Fiona writes, "*A few weeks ago little Eric, from Atlanta, GA, developed a nasty bout of impetigo. His mother was really worried because she couldn't get hold of any antibiotics to calm it down and they were having a BBQ that day with lots of his friends invited. I really wanted something to help immediately, and a friend said she had just purchased some allicin capsules and a small supply of liquid. We used it immediately on Eric and, within a few hours, the attack had subsided and his sores began to clear up. We were naturally delighted and would recommend this to anyone else who suffers from this debilitating condition.*"

IMPOTENCE

Allicin can increase the production of nitric oxide sythase, which is vital for maintaining a healthy blood supply to the penis. No work has yet been published specifically regarding the effect of stabilized allicin on impotence, but it's well worth a try!

IRRITABLE BOWEL SYNDROME

Medical definition

This is a common condition in which recurrent abdominal pain with constipation and/or diarrhea continues for years without any deterioration in general health. Although the cause is unknown, it is generally accepted that stress, anxiety and a series of recurrent infections in the intestine all contribute to IBS.

Most doctors now agree that people who suffer from a wide range of digestive problems are likely to have an imbalance in the quality and content of their intestinal flora. Our stomach contains many hundreds of bacterial species, some of which are aggressive to our digestive system but many that are absolutely necessary for maintaining a normal, healthy, functioning digestive system. When, for whatever reason, this balance is upset, symptoms will occur, and until the balance is reset, many people will suffer consistently.

Allicin can be described as a prebiotic in that it possesses an ability to kill harmful digestive bacteria like *Salmonella* and *Escherichia coli,* but will leave healthy bacterial species like *Lactobacillus* and *Acidopholus* alone. This means that your own population of friendly bacteria can go about their business and continue to flourish and replicate without any problems from an over-population of nasty bugs. If you add a good quality probiotic (pick one that is multi-strain and offers as many friendly bacterial strains as possible), you will also add significantly to your friendly digestive population. Within a very short period of time, you will notice that your bowel habits return to normal and that you can happily eat whatever you like.

Treatment regimen

Add 2-4 capsules of allicin plus a multi-strain probiotic to every meal. A balanced probiotic that can provide a large number of "friendly" bacteria should be used.

Testimonial

Jenny B from Stone in Kent has never been able to digest certain foods, especially bread. Already a convert to allicin, she added in a probiotic and followed the regimen detailed above. Within just a matter of days, she was able to digest meals more easily. Bread no longer gave her stomach cramps or constipation.

LEISHMANIASIS

Leishmaniasis is a disease common in the tropics and sub-tropics caused by parasitic protozoans of the genus, leishmania, which is transmitted by the bite of sandflies. There are two principal forms of the disease: visceral leishmaniais, in which the cells of various internal organs are affected, and cutaneous leishmaniasis which affects the tissues of the skin. The latter has several different forms depending on the region in which it occurs and the protozoal species involved. Countries such as Panama, Honduras, the Amazon, South Central America and Asia are areas where leismaniaisis is the most common.

❝ Allicin liquid is a natural anti-parasitic agent that has been recently shown to kill head lice after just two applications.❞

In Asia, this appears in the form of a sore and can be seen as a major-third world problem. Leishmaniasis is a disease of the skin and mucous membranes, resulting in ulcerating lesions found on the arms and legs. The infection may also spread to the mucous membranes of the nose and mouth, causing serious destruction of the tissues. Standard treatment is normally with drugs containing antimony, but these are generally not readily available or well tolerated.

A form of leishmaniaisis of the skin caused by the parasite, *leishmania tropica mexicana,* is also known as Chiclero's ulcer. The disease which occurs in Panama, Honduras and the Amazon, primarily affects men who visit the forests to collect chicle (gum).

This condition takes the form of an ulcerating lesion on the ear lobe. Although the sore usually heals spontaneously within 6 months, it can cause a great deal of discomfort.

Kala-azar (visceral leishmaniasis) or Dumdum fever is another common form, which occurs in Asia, South America, and the Mediterranean area of Africa. Symptoms include enlargement of the liver and spleen, anemia, weight loss and fever.

Allicin liquid is a natural anti-parasitic agent that has been recently shown to kill head lice after just two applications. The compound has also shown exceptional antibiotic and antiviral activity. *In vitro* tests at the University of East London using allicin liquid have also shown very promising results in eradicating these protozoal parasites.

Treatment regimen

A combination of treatment with allicin liquid and/or creme applied to any ulceration that develops will help to remove infection. Apply as often as necessary, but initially, at least 3 times a day to the affected area. At the same time, it is vital to get enough allicin into the bloodstream to force any parasites out of the body. The holistic approach of "heal from within and from without" applies especially to leishmaniasis, so take at least 6 allicin powder capsules per day for at least 2 months.

MOLLUSCUM CONTAGIOSUM

Medical definition

This is a common disease of the skin, mainly affecting children. Characterized by papules less than 5mm in diameter, each with a central depression, the disease is caused by a pox virus (others in this group include variola responsible for smallpox and vaccinia which causes cowpox) and is spread by direct contact. Untreated, the papules will disappear within 2 years.

This is a very distressing and unpleasant disease found in children, especially those starting preschool. Most doctors will say that you just have to let the disease run its natural course. Well, now we have allicin! Please read the testimonial below as it really sums up how good allicin can be.

Testimonial and Treatment regimen

Earlier this year I was told by our doctor that our daughter was suffering from Molluscum Contagiosum, a condition of the skin that causes wart-like spots which eventually (over a period of months or even years) turn into large and painful pustules which eventually burst, sometimes leaving behind a scar or pit. She was five years old at the time, and we had first noticed some spots when she was only two. Gradually, over this time, they had spread from her trunk and arms to her legs, and particularly between her legs and around the genital area.

They were causing her a great deal of discomfort and embarrassment, so it was most distressing to hear from the doctor that there was absolutely no treatment for them because they were caused by a virus. We were told that although painful and unsightly, they were otherwise totally harmless and that they would disappear eventually.

When I heard, through a friend, that it may be possible to treat them with garlic, I decided that anything was worth a try. Apparently, garlic has anti-viral properties (among many other benefits including anti-bacterial and anti-fungal). Through the Garlic Information Centre, we were given a bottle of allicin liquid (a component of fresh garlic most associated with healing properties) and told to apply it to our daughter's spots twice a day with a cotton bud.

After only three days there was a noticeable improvement, and after a week the spots had completely gone. We were absolutely thrilled and could hardly believe that allicin had worked so effectively and so quickly!

I know from talking to other parents that Molluscum Contagiosum is common in young children and that it seems to be particularly rife at the moment, not just in my area, but countrywide. I would thoroughly recommend trying this treatment. It can do no harm and may work for others as it has for us!

Claudia Macpherson, United Kingdom

MOSQUITOES
Medical definition

A small, winged, blood-sucking insect belonging to a large group—the Diptera—or two-winged flies. Its mouthparts are formed into a long proboscis for piercing the skin and sucking blood. Female mosquitoes transmit the parasites responsible for several major infectious diseases, including malaria and West Nile virus.

Mosquitoes can be found all over the world from the tropics to the Arctic. Some mosquitoes can be found 200 miles from their birthplace. One species of *Anopheles* frequently becomes frozen, but after gradual thawing, revives and is capable of laying eggs. Of all the harmful creatures on earth, this little "vampire" probably poses the greatest threat to mankind. There are more than 3,450 species in the culicid or mosquito family worldwide, and mosquito-borne diseases infect about 700 million people each year, killing 3 million according to the Centers for Disease Control. The US and Canada spend about $150 million each year trying to *control* mosquitoes with poison. Residents spend more than that on repellents, insecticide poisons, screens and other products in the vain attempt to *control* mosquitoes. Only the females bite and then only when they are actively reproducing.

By 1995, at least 1 of 4 species of the Plasmodium parasite that infect humans, e.g., *Plasmodium vivax*, *Plasmodium falciparum*, *Plasmodium malariae* and *Plasmodium ovale*, were found living in the blood of nearly 300 million people. Malaria is transferred to humans only via mosquitoes and now affects 300 - 500 million new people per year, killing 1.5 to 2.7 million people per year. Quinine no longer can control malaria, because the disease has developed resistance to it. Malaria is found in at least 102 countries. In 395 A.D., 330,000 acres of farmland in Rome's Compania region were abandoned due to a malaria epidemic.

Mosquitoes are blood-feeding ectoparasites of people and animals. The English call mosquitoes "gnats" and the Scottish call them "midges." Malaria is caused by the presence of parasitic protozoa of the genus *Plasmodium*, which are deposited into red blood cells by the biting female mosquito. Parasites found within the red blood cells and liver cells of humans are taken into the stomach of the mosquito as it feeds, where they multiply and invade the salivary glands. When the mosquito bites an individual, parasites are injected into the bloodstream.

There are about 100 trillion mosquitoes with at least 3,450 different species in the world. Morphologically, mosquito males differ from females in that they have feathery antennae, long feathery palps and smaller mouthparts. Mosquitoes develop through complete metamorphosis and have four distinct states: egg, larva or "wriggler," pupa or "tumbler" and adult.

Mosquito eggs can be classified into three groups:

- Eggs laid singly on the still or very slow-moving water surface (*Anopheles*), with each egg having a series of "floats" along its perimeter
- Eggs laid in groups forming rafts, made by the adult females, that float on water surfaces (*Culex and Culiseta*) and
- Eggs laid singly out of the water in the mud (*Aedes and Psorophora*)

Mosquito larvae are aquatic; they feed on water mites, water fleas, algae, protozoans and minute organic debris by sweeping the food into their mouths with a pair of feeding brushes. Mosquito pupae also live in the water. Adult mosquitoes are small, about 1/8" long, with a single pair of membranous wings and are free living. A typical mosquito weights about 2.5 milligrams, or about 20,000 mosquitoes per pound. Males do not feed as adults, but females of most species require a human and/or animal blood meal before oviposition, utilizing the protein in blood to produce their eggs and bring them to maturity.

Mosquitoes seriously harm vast numbers of people worldwide by transmitting pathogenic organisms that cause disease and death, especially in tropical areas. This includes eastern and western states particularly California and Missouri where malaria is a constant threat where known vectors exist. Malaria, among all insect-borne diseases, has been the most deadly in modern history. During this century alone it has killed between 100-300 million people, mostly babies and small children and it infects and debilitates hundreds of millions of others each year. It has been suggested by CNN that 700,000,000 people a year are infected, with a disease carried by mosquitoes.

"There are an estimated 10 trillion mosquitoes produced just in the U. S. each summer."

In Canada hordes of mosquitoes can actually darken the sky - researchers were bitten about 9,000 times per minute; at that rate they could lose 1/2 their blood in 2 hours and die from blood loss! But our primary reason for controlling mosquitoes usually is only to lessen the annoyance caused by their bites and secondarily to reduce the transmission of human and equine viral encephalitis and dog heartworm. The annoyance caused by mosquito feeding can include the itching, restlessness, loss of sleep and nervous irritation in all people, pets and domestic animals that suffer from their attacks. Mosquitoes do not really "bite," but they penetrate their victim's hide or skin with their proboscis or hollow, flexible snout. The female has a pump in her head which she uses like a turkey baster to suck in your blood. The average meal takes about 1 millionth of a gallon per bite. Their saliva makes us itch. Usually this *minor* annoyance cannot be documented in terms of economic loss, but, obviously, there may be some major economic losses, e.g., decreased recreation income and lower milk and beef production due to blood loss and irritation. Occasionally extremely

large numbers of mosquitoes can actually cause the death of domestic animals through blood loss and anaphylactic shock from reactions to mass injections of mosquito saliva. Mosquitoes are not strong flyers- so fans easily blow them away.
There are an estimated 10 trillion mosquitoes produced just in the U.S. each summer with about 170 species. To give you some idea how many 10 trillion is—it amounts to 41,000 mosquitoes for every man, woman and child in America or enough to fill the entire Grand Canyon! A mosquito's brain is the size of the full stop at the end of this sentence, yet it has outwitted man since the dawn of recorded history.

"When travelling it is important to ensure you get as much allicin in your bloodstream as possible."

What can garlic and allicin do to help?
The surface features of the eggs of *Aedes aegypti (L.)* and the effect of garlic extracts on their hatching were studied by scanning electron microscopy. The exochorion and endochorion layers of the eggshells display an essentially pentagonal reticulation. The exochorion meshwork exhibits large and small papillae interconnected by horizontal struts. At higher magnification, the large papillae show aeropyles on their rough surface. Eggs hatched in deionized water undergo complete fracture near the anterior poles producing free shell caps. In contrast, eggs placed in 6% reconstituted aged garlic extract are only partially fractured, display attached shell caps, and the larvae remain trapped within the shells. In the natural garlic bulb extract, the eggs show no fracture lines in their shells. No larvae were observed either alive or dead in the garlic extracts, suggesting the embryos were disabled before they could escape from their eggshells as viable larvae. It is concluded that

aqueous extracts of garlic inhibit hatching of Aedes eggs. Thus, compounds in garlic may be beneficial in the control of mosquitoes.

Treatment regimen

Take 6-10 allicin powder capsules every day for at least 1 month and then reduce this back down to 2 per day. At the same time take allicin liquid and dilute it with distilled water: 1 part allicin liquid to 1 part water and take this 3 times per day for at least 1 month. Also, immediately apply a few drops of liquid to any bites that you get. This will reduce inflammation and pain whilst allowing the wound to heal much faster.

When traveling it is important to ensure you get as much allicin in your bloodstream as possible, although it is important to point out that we have had several reports of people who completely avoided being bitten on just 1 capsule per day!

If you have areas in the yard where water lies then it would also be sensible during the summer months to consider diluting some allicin liquid and spraying onto the water to prevent the eggs from developing. Again a 1 to 3 dilution will be sufficient.

Testimonials

Mr. B Groom from London, England took part in a study to confirm the antiviral properties of allicin powder, he went on holiday to Egypt with a party of friends who were not taking the capsules. Everyone around him got bitten by mosquitoes but he did not get bitten once.

Mrs. CM from Florida reports that she has used allicin liquid applied directly to a number of mosquito bites and they calmed down almost immediately.

Mr. JF also from Florida has used the liquid diluted into water and sprayed onto his horses to prevent attacks from mosquitoes. "*It worked really well just by spraying 2-3 times a day. I diluted the allicin liquid 1 part to 3 with water. My horses actually seemed to like it!*"

Mr. NB from Rye in Sussex, England performed a very interesting experiment in a trough of water in his backyard. He noticed a number of small adult mosquitoes feeding in the water and on the surface. Taking some allicin liquid concentrate he simply added a few drops (about 20 drops) to the water and stirred it around. Over the next few days the adult flies were seen floating on the surface of the water having been killed and subsequently no larvae hatched.

MRSA INFECTION
Methicillin resistant Staphylococcus aureus—The SUPERBUG!
Headlines in newspapers around the world state:
"Superbug strain hits the healthy"
"Superbug hits 11,000 patients on dirty wards"
"One patient in 10 gets a hospital bug"
"Cases of deadly hospital superbug hit 200 a week"
"Twenty-three-year-old dies of MRSA after routine operation"
and one headline that may offer some hope—
"Garlic creme beats hospital superbugs"

What is MRSA?
Staphylococcus is a family of common bacteria.

Many people naturally carry it in their throats and nasal cavities, and it can cause a mild infection in a healthy patient. MRSA stands for methicillin-resistant *Staphylococcus aureus*, but is shorthand for any strain of Staphylococcus bacteria, which is resistant to one or more conventional antibiotics.

There are many different strains of MRSA, with differing degrees of immunity to the effects of various antibiotics.

It doesn't mean that antibiotics are completely powerless against it. It may simply require a much higher dose over a much longer period, or the use of an alternative antibiotic to which the bug has less resistance.

Why does MRSA exist?

It's all about survival of the fittest—the basic principle of evolution, and bacteria have been around a lot longer than us, so they're pretty good at it.

There are countless strains of a single type of bacteria, and each has subtle natural genetic mutations, which make it different from the other. In addition, bacterial genes are constantly mutating. Some strains' genetic makeup will give them a slight advantage when it comes to fighting off antibiotic attack. So when weaker strains encounter antibiotics, they die, while these naturally resistant strains may prove harder to kill. This means that next time you encounter *Staph*, it is more likely to be one which has survived an antibiotic encounter, i.e., a resistant one.

The advice from doctors who prescribe antibiotics is always to finish the entire course—advice which many of us ignore.

When you don't finish the course, there's a chance that you'll kill most of the bugs, but not all of them and the ones that survive are, of course, likely to be those that are most resistant to antibiotics.

Over time, the bulk of the Staph strains will carry resistance genes, and further mutations may only add to their survival ability. Strains that manage to carry two or three resistance genes will have extraordinary powers of resistance to antibiotics.

"Doctors are very worried about what the future holds for MRSA."

The reason that hospitals seem to be hotbeds for resistant MRSA is because so many different strains are being thrown together with so many doses of antibiotics, vastly accelerating this natural selection process.

Why is it so dangerous?

It is a fact of life that patients are at higher than normal risk of picking up a Staph infection on the wards of any hospital anywhere in the world. This is for two reasons. First, that the population in hospitals tends to be older, sicker and weaker than the general population, making them more vulnerable to the infection.

Second, conditions in hospitals, which involve a great many people living cheek by jowl, examined by doctors and nurses who have just touched other patients, are the perfect environment for the transmission of all manner of infections. Staph infections can be dangerous in weakened patients, particularly if they can't be cleared up quickly with antibiotic treatments. MRSA infections can prove tough to treat because they are resistant to treatment, making them more dangerous than a simple case of Staph.

What is likely to happen in the future?

Doctors are very worried about what the future holds for MRSA.

The number of reports of MRSA infections rises year by year and the latest evidence suggests that deaths due to MRSA are increasing at a similar rate. Already, the spectre of a bug resistant to all antibiotics is approaching. VRSA, or vancomycin resistant *Staphylococcus Aureus*, has acquired resistance to a drug considered the "last line of defence" when all other antibiotics have failed.

The UK has already seen several cases of GISA, or glycopeptide intermediate resistant *Staphylococcus aureus*, a kind of "halfway house" between MRSA and VRSA, which has developed a resistance to antibiotics of the vancomycin family.

Although new antibiotics are being developed all the time, pessimistic experts believe it is only a matter of time until virtually every weapon in the pharmaceutical arsenal is nullified.

Nihilists suggest that there could come a point at which bacteria retake the upper hand, and doctors, as in previous centuries, have no answer to some bacterial infections.

It should be noted, they say, that humans have only had the upper hand over bacteria for a handful of decades. We have no right to expect that situation to last forever.

What can we do about it now?

The government is already trying to at least slow down the apparently relentless march of the bacteria. One of the main reasons behind their swift evolution into "superbugs" is the overuse of antibiotics, both in human and veterinary medicine. Until recently, patients visiting their doctor with a viral infection might demand, and be given an antibiotic prescription—despite the fact that antibiotics have no effect on this.

All those patients were doing was strengthening the communities of bacteria in their bodies.

Doctors have now been told to cut antibiotic prescribing.

Hygiene is another tried and tested way of at least protecting the most vulnerable patients from the most dangerous strains.

Handwashing between patients should be a must for doctors and nurses, or they are simply doing more harm than good in their trips around the wards.

Ministers are trying to improve overall standards of hygiene, perhaps by reintroducing the concept of the ward matron, with responsibility for cleanliness.

But more frighteningly in recent months (March 2003), reports from California suggest that MRSA is now beginning to infect thousands of people across America and Europe. It is now a fact that a new strain is emerging that spreads through skin contact and can even infect healthy people. US-CDC in Atlanta stated, "We are greatly concerned that MRSA has emerged into the healthy population." The strain has been spreading like wildfire in crowded jails and across cities and towns all over the United States. Athletes, schoolchildren, homosexuals and newborns have all fallen victim to this superbug. The infection usually appears as sores that resemble insect bites and nasty boils and abcesses can develop usually requiring repeated courses of antibiotics and sometimes surgery. The worry is that it could reach the lungs or bloodstream where it could cause pneumonia or septicaemia. The scary possibility is that with all these extra antibiotics being dished out like peas, we could be only weeks away from developing a multi-drug resistant strain. There has even been one report of this superbug spreading via food and causing gastroenteritis. Further reports show that the gay community could be facing another onslaught of deadly microbial disease since this bug is also infecting HIV negative men as well as those who already have the HIV virus.

Whether a dirty ward rather than a dirty hand is a reservoir for Staphylococcus is a matter of debate, however. In the long run, many experts suggest it may take a breakthrough akin to the discovery of penicillin before humans can regain a temporary upper hand over the bugs again—and this is precisely where we stand TODAY WITH ALLICIN.

Take a look at the chart and you will see that allicin liquid, powder and creme can ALL kill multiple strains of MRSA at a concentration as low as 250ppm allicin. Indeed every batch of allicin formulations that are produced are now tested against an MRSA bacterium and every time billions of bacteria are wiped out with allicin.

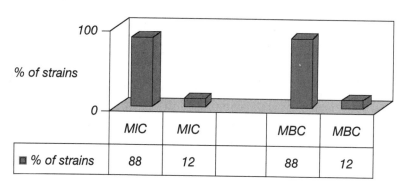

Mininimum inhibitory (MIC) and Minimum Bactericidal (MBC) Concentrations for Allicin (μg/ml) against Clinical isolates of Staphylococcus aureus

	MIC	MIC		MBC	MBC
■ % of strains	88	12		88	12

Allicin liquid and allicin creme offers a third option

Currently, in hospitals around the world, there are only 2 pharmaceutical agents that have any chance of killing MRSA. One is vancomycin, usually given intravenously. (But very worryingly an oral version is now available and is dished out to anyone who goes home from hospital after developing a wound infection. Remember, most people put onto oral antibiotics never finish the course and this can lead to the development of resistant strains of bacteria.) The other is a cream for topical use called mupirocin. This particular agent has also now seen *Staphylococcus aureus* develop a large number of resistant strains and mupirocin is proving to be less effective than at any time since its launch in the 1970s.

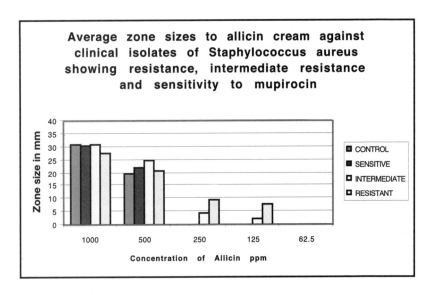

Work is now underway to prove that allicin creme, and a special powder combination, when placed into the nasal cavity can kill MRSA. This will give 2 methods for treating infected healthcare workers. With the ongoing development of allicin soap to help prevent the passage of infection between staff and patients this will give a genuine third option for hospitals, rest homes, nursing homes and other institutions where MRSA is common.

Interestingly, our research so far seems to indicate that the drug resistant species of *Staphylococcus aureus* are the easiest to kill with allicin liquid powder and creme. This means that microbiologists will have the capability to use a safe, natural and effective plant derived antibacterial agent. Certainly in the UK, the problem is very significant with EVERY district general hospital in a recent survey indicating a serious problem with MRSA infected wards. Most hospitals worldwide do not know how many staff actually carry MRSA in their noses. It is, at least for them, better not to know.

Patients now get released from hospitals too soon, even before wounds have properly healed. Speaking with my own doctor recently, he could name 8 patients in our local area who had a resistant MRSA infection at home trying departely to get rid of it. One such person was Deborah whose own case history she reports below.

Testimonial

Deborah's wounds are on her spine. One close to the top, which is approx. 2cm by 1.5cm. This is overgranulated and weeps. The other is approx. 0.75cm by 0.5cm and near her waistline. This is overgranulated but only weeps a little. She had a major spinal operation two years ago and although she has had antibiotics through a Hickman line and a wash-out so far nothing has worked. She has been on oral antibiotics and creams for several months but nothing has been able to shift the infection (it's called MRSA). The only option now available to her via the hospital is to have all the metalwork [in her spine] removed. As you can imagine she does not want to go back into the hospital nor does she want the metalwork removed. We would be very grateful if you could produce a cream and some capsules for her. If you require any further information we can speak to the district nurses on Saturday. They dress her wounds then whilst I do them during the week.
Just a few weeks later—
Dear Peter,

I had not been in touch as mum said she had emailed you. I don't think she wanted to get carried away, but the news is very exciting. I no longer have any infection in my back and it is all thanks to the treatments you so generously suggested. Having had these two wounds on my back weeping for 2 years I don't know quite how to thank you and hope that I get the opportunity to thank you in person at some point. I will also be telling anyone who may benefit from allicin how miraculous it is.

I am going to the hospital on Thursday. I am not sure if my consultant can quite believe what has happened, as he, along with some of my district nurses, are not too happy about the thought of using alternative remedies. When I think how many courses of antibiotics I have been instructed to take in the last 2 years and how many biopsies came back positive for MRSA, I am not surprised that the medical staff cannot believe it!

The new scented cream sounds great, although I have plenty at the minute. I am running out of capsules, but know where I can buy them.

Thank you once again for all you have done. You saved me from another horrendous operation. Maybe I can repay you in some way. For instance, if it would be of any benefit, I could write something about my experience with MRSA and how allicin cured it, if that might help promote the product—just a thought.

Yours eternally grateful,

Deborah

The following "plate pictures" show just how effective allicin is at combatting MRSA. My thanks to Dr. Ron Cutler at the University of East London for the pictures.

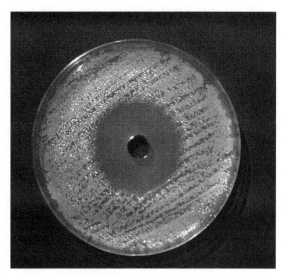

Allicin Liquid – Zone of inhibition produced by allicin against MRSA103

The above shows quite clearly that allicin liquid can kill billions of nasty MRSA bacteria. The two other plate pictures show how much more effective allicin creme is than the only topical agent currently used in hospitals and in the community worldwide—mupirocin.

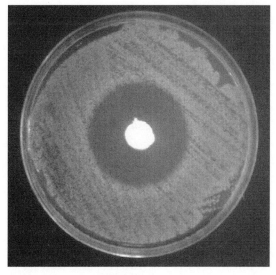

Allicin Creme

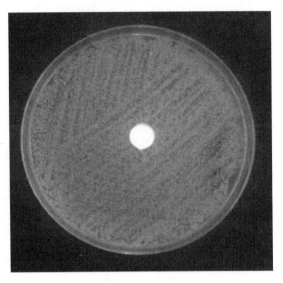

Mupirocin Creme
Allicin creme (previous page) compared with mupirocin (above) against MRSA.
Clearly shows superiority in favour of allicin as a topical treatment for MRSA infections
on the skin and in the nasal cavity.

PARASITES

Medical definition

Any living thing, that lives in or on another living organism. The parasite, which may spend all or only part of its existence with the host, obtains food and/or shelter from the host and contributes nothing to its welfare. Some parasites cause irritation and interfere with bodily functions. Others destroy host tissues and release toxins into the body, thus injuring health and causing disease.

Human parasites, including fungi, bacteria, viruses, protozoa and worms, can all be treated with allicin.

Antiparasitic properties of allicin

The antiparasitic effects of freshly crushed garlic were known by many ancient cultures. Albert Schweizer used to treat people suffering from dysentery or intestinal worms with freshly crushed garlic. One of the traditional Chinese medical treatments for intestinal diseases is an alcoholic extract of crushed garlic cloves. Several years ago it was noted that *Entamoeba histolytica*, the human intestinal protozoan parasite, is very sensitive to allicin, as only 300 parts per million of allicin totally inhibits the growth of these amoeba cultures. More recent data shows that at lower concentrations (30 parts per million), allicin inhibits 90% of the virulence of trophozoites of *Enantamoeba Histolytica*.

Allicin also very efficiently inhibits the growth of other protozoan parasites, such as *Giardia lamblia, Leishmania major, Leptomonas colosoma*, and *Crithidia fasciculata*. Interestingly, at high allicin concentrations no damage to the mammalian cells is seen, suggesting that the affinity of the allicin molecules is towards the parasite targets.

The AIDS Research Alliance in California has been testing the effectiveness of allicin in combating cryptosporidiosis, a parasitic infection of the intestinal tract. The tests involved patients taking liquid allicin mixed with distilled water twice daily. Patients suffered from less diarrhea and had stable or increasing body weight. For several patients, repeated testing showed negative results for cryptosporidium parasites. Larger trials are planned. Allicin in combination with agents, such as black walnut hulls, wormwood, grapefruit seed extract, cloves and gentian would make an ideal antiparasite formulation.

Treatment regimen

Take 6 allicin powder capsules every day for at least 1 month and then reduce this back down to 2 per day. At the same time take allicin liquid and dilute it with distilled water: 1 part allicin liquid to 1 part water and take this 3 times per day for at least 1 month.

PARONYCHIA
Medical definition
An inflamed swelling of the nail folds usually caused by infection with Staphylococcus aureus. *Chronic paronychia usually occurs in those who habitually engage in wet work where a secondary infection is caused by* Candida albicans.

Antibiotics are often prescribed, but the bacteria is now multi-drug resistant and therefore you must use an agent like allicin that can kill both a bacterial and fungal infection. These two particular organisms are the most sensitive to allicin liquid and powder formulations—meaning they are easily destroyed by allicin.

Treatment regimen
Apply allicin liquid directly to the infected area. Just a few drops per day will be needed. Take 2-4 allicin capsules every day to get rid of any systemic infection (this is very common with Candida) and continue to take them after the infection clears to prevent it from returning.

PEPTIC ULCER
Medical definition
This is a breach in the lining of the digestive tract caused by digestion of the mucosa by pepsin and acid. A peptic ulcer can be found in the esophagus, the stomach, duodenum or jejunum.

Ulcers are incredibly common and for many years the medical profession had been convinced that the main cause was an overproduction of stomach acid. However, we now know that even people with low volumes of stomach acid can get ulcers and stomach cancer is actually very common in people who cannot produce ANY stomach acid (achlorhydria) at all.

It has now been established that upwards of 50% of the population of the entire world carry an infectious organism in their stomach. Called

Helicobacter pylori, this is a spiral shaped bacterium that lives in the stomach and duodenum (section of intestine just below stomach). It has a unique way of adapting in the harsh environment of the stomach. The inside of the stomach is bathed in about half a gallon of gastric juice every day. Gastric juice is composed of digestive enzymes and concentrated hydrochloric acid, which can readily tear apart the toughest food or microorganism. Bacteria, viruses, and yesterday's steak dinner are all consumed in this deadly bath of chemicals. It used to be thought that the stomach contained no bacteria and was actually sterile, but *Helicobacter pylori* changed that. It is often described as an acid-fast bacterium and it loves your stomach acid.

The stomach is protected from its own gastric juice by a thick layer of mucus that covers the stomach lining. *Helicobacter pylori* takes advantage of this protection by living in the mucus lining. Once the bacterium is safely ensconced in the mucus, it is able to fight the stomach acid that does reach it with an enzyme it possesses called urease. Urease converts urea, of which there is an abundant supply in the stomach (from saliva and gastric juices), into bicarbonate and ammonia, which are strong bases. This creates a cloud of acid neutralizing chemicals around the *Helicobacter pylori,* protecting it from the acid in the stomach. The reaction of urea hydrolysis is important for diagnosis of *Helicobacter pylori* by the breath test.

Another protective mechanism that *Helicobacter* has is that the body's natural defenses cannot reach the bacterium in the mucus lining of the stomach. The immune system will respond to an *H. pylori* infection by sending white cells, killer T cells, and other infection-fighting agents. However, these potential *H. pylori* eradicators cannot reach the infection, because they cannot easily get through the stomach lining. Naturally, allicin will boost the number of T cells available to your immune system and enable a stronger reaction to this invasive organism to be produced. This will mean that the immune response grows and grows. Polymorphs die, and spill their destructive compounds (superoxide radicals) on stomach lining cells. Extra nutrients are sent to reinforce the white cells, and the *H. pylori* can feed on this. Within a few days, gastritis and perhaps eventually a peptic ulcer results. It may not be *H. pylori* itself which causes peptic ulcer, but the inflammation of the stomach lining; i.e., the response to *H. pylori*.

But here is the bad news. *Helicobacter pylori* is believed to be transmitted *orally*. Many researchers think that *Helicobacter pylori* is transmitted orally by means of fecal matter through the ingestion of waste tainted food or water. In addition, it is possible that the infection could be transmitted from the stomach to the mouth through gastro-esophagal reflux (in which a small amount of the stomach's contents is involuntarily forced up the esophagus) or belching, common symptoms of gastritis. The bacterium could then be transmitted through oral contact. So you must consider protecting yourself from a repeat infection by taking a regular dose of allicin powder capsules.

Treatment of *Helicobacter pylori* infection is difficult and there is a small risk associated with taking bismuth drugs (for example, Pepto-Bismol). They may temporarily cause gray staining of the teeth and mouth and can cause constipation, diarrhea, and blackening of the stools. All antibiotics have a small risk of an allergic reaction and have a list of side effects as long as your arm. The antibiotics recommended are called amoxycillin, clarithromycin, tetracycline. ALL of these antibiotics will work better if you take allicin powder capsules at the same time, since allicin has an ability to work synergistically with a wide range of pharmaceutical agents. This means that you should need less drug if you add allicin powder capsules into your treatment regimen. If your *Helicobacter pylori* infection is difficult to cure, you may need to take a large dose of allicin all in one go (see treatment regimen below).

We estimate that allicin can kill *Helicobacter pylori* at a concentration of just 16ppm and every powdered capsule has a minimum concentration of 300ppm allicin! Several studies published over the last few years have shown that water based extracts of garlic can kill this organism very easily. Remember that allicin is produced as a water-based liquid that is conventionally spray dried so it has activity against this nasty bacterium.

Treatment regimen

You will need to take a relatively large dose of allicin over a 2-4 week period to prevent the release of urea and to enable the allicin to penetrate the protective lining of the stomach so as to seek and destroy the Helicobacter infection. Take 6-10 capsules every day either all in one go or you can spread them out over the day. If you are already on a course of antibiotics, this dose should be cut in half. If the combination doesn't clear the infection, try using just allicin at the increased dosage level.

PREGNANCY – PRE-ECLAMPSIA
Medical definition

This is a high blood pressure developed during pregnancy in women whose BP was usually normal.

It is important to try to get the patient under control as quickly as possible, since a high blood pressure can have serious consequences for both the baby and the mother. Early work suggests that allicin may play a significant role in the prevention of pre-eclampsia and it is perfectly safe to take. This is in direct opposition to the use of pharmaceutical agents, which can rarely be used in pregnancy for fear of a serious direct affect on the baby.

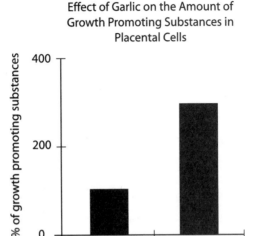

Effect of Garlic on the Amount of Growth Promoting Substances in Placental Cells

Research shows that taking allicin during pregnancy can cut the risk of pre-eclampsia (raised blood pressure and protein retained in the urine). Studies reveal that allicin may help to boost the birthweight of babies otherwise destined to be too small.

The research was carried out by Dr. D. Sooranna, Ms J. Hirani and Dr. I. Das in the Academic Department of Obstetrics & Gynaecology at the Chelsea & Westminster Hospital in London, UK. They concluded that although pre-eclampsia and growth retardation are complex conditions, with a variety of known and unknown causes, taking a standardised allicin concentration throughout pregnancy may decrease the chances of these types of complications at birth. They focused on growth-retarded babies and pre-eclampsia, a potentially dangerous condition for mother and baby, which occurs in about one in ten pregnancies. Experiments by the research team showed that adding extracts of allicin to cells from the placenta of women likely to suffer from these conditions was able to quickly stimulate growth. Furthermore, the activity of key enzymes that are reduced in abnormal pregnancies were significantly increased when allicin was added.

Treatment regimen

Just one capsule a day should be taken throughout the pregnancy but this can be doubled or tripled if the blood pressure starts to rise. Several "mums" with a history of pre-eclampsia have used allicin during pregnancy and have not reported any rise in blood pressure.

PROTOZOAL INFECTIONS

See parasites

PSORIASIS

Medical definition

Psoriasis is a chronic, but treatable autoimmune skin disease experienced by an estimated 5-6 million Americans and about 80 million people around the world.

While psoriasis is not typically life-threatening, it can greatly affect your appearance, self-esteem and overall quality of life. It can develop anywhere on the skin, though it usually appears on the scalp, knees, elbows and torso. It may also affect the nails and joints.

Psoriasis of the skin has several common symptoms. It is often itchy and may cause painful drying, cracking or blistering of the skin. Psoriasis affecting the joints (psoriatic arthritis) can cause pain and make movement more difficult.

Red, raised areas of skin called plaques characterize plaque psoriasis are the most common form of the disease. Plaque psoriasis can range from mild to severe. Approximately 20 to 25 percent of cases are severe. Other forms of the disease include guttate psoriasis, erythrodermic psoriasis and pustular psoriasis.

Many people with psoriasis develop it in their 20s, but the disease can occur at any age, even childhood. It is equally common in men and women, and tends to run in families. Treatments for psoriasis include the use of skin creams, light therapy, and systemic therapies (pills or injections).

The exact causes of psoriasis are complex and not fully understood, but genetic traits leading to abnormalities in the body's response to infection are believed to be the underlying basis. A specialized type of white blood cell called a T cell has been identified as playing a key role in the inflammation that eventually leads to psoriasis plaques and related symptoms.

Although scientists have not yet identified the exact cause or causes of psoriasis, they do know that psoriasis begins in the body's immune system. Specifically, it is triggered when a certain type of T cell malfunctions and reproduces uncontrollably. These malfunctioning T cells travel to the surface of the skin and start an inflammatory reaction in which skin cells multiply 7 to 12 times faster than normal. The end result is the formation of psoriatic plaques. Allicin treatment for psoriasis fights back by reaching far beneath the skin to halt this psoriatic process exactly where it starts—in the immune system.

There also appears to be a genetic component to the disease, which tends to run in families. Statistically speaking, 30 to 50 percent of people with psoriasis have relatives with the disease. A child born to two parents who have psoriasis is more likely to develop it than if one parent has psoriasis; the risk also is high—but not 100 percent—if an identical twin has psoriasis, which suggests that genes alone are not responsible.

Environmental factors are thought to trigger an attack in people who have a genetic tendency toward the disease. The environment may also cause flare-ups, which are the periods when existing skin plaques worsen temporarily. Flares are common in psoriasis, as are remissions, when the disease appears to get better suddenly.

Several triggers have been linked to psoriasis flares, including:

- **Damage to the skin** – Injury, frequent rubbing or scratching the skin may cause plaques to worsen in a process known as Koebner's phenomenon.
- **Infections** – Streptococcal throat infections (strep throat) may trigger guttate psoriasis, a form of psoriasis that usually occurs in childhood.
- **Medications** – Drugs linked to a worsening of psoriasis include lithium, drugs used to treat malaria, beta blockers, non-steroidal anti inflammatory drugs, and oral steroids.
- **Stress** – Some studies have linked stress to flares, which can occur as much as one month after the stressful event.
- **Stapylococccal infections** normally resident in the nasal cavity of nonsufferers are much more common in psoriasis sufferers on various parts of the body (see table below). In some instances more than a twenty-fold increase in Staph carriage. This bacterial species has become multi-drug resistant and its presence in psoriatic plaques will lead to a secondary infection and a worsening of clinical symptoms.

Percentage prevelance of Staphylococcus aureus infection	Normal individuals	Psoriasis sufferers
NOSE	34	37
CHEEK	7	16
CHEST	3	21
FOREARM	2	16
SCAPULA	2	37

Table showing percentage carriage of Staphylococcus aureus *in normal individuals and psoriasis sufferers.*

- **Alcohol and smoking** – Drinking and smoking are not considered major risk factors for developing psoriasis, but they may trigger flares, especially alcohol consumption in men and smoking in women.
- **Diet** – While nutrition may play a role in psoriasis, the scientific basis for improving symptoms with diet has not been established.
- **Climate** – Psoriasis is often better in the summer months, when the skin is exposed to sunshine, and worse during the cloudy winter months. Winter may be a good time for a vacation to a sunny spot!

Treatment regimen

Allicin powder capsules, creme and liquid formulations can offer two major benefits for psoriasis sufferers. First, by boosting the immune system and stimulating the production of normal T cells. This will enable the body to fight off the over-production of malfunctioning cells. Next by removing the invasive bacterial infections, whether they be staph or strep species.

Take 2-6 allicin powder capsules per day and treat any plaques with creme or liquid twice daily.

RINGWORM

Medical definition

This is a fungal infection of the skin, scalp and nails. Caused by dermatophyte Microsporium trichophyton and Epidermaphyton which can affect animals and they are usually the source of infection in man. Can be spread by direct contact or by infected materials. Lesions are ring-like and cause intense itching. Ringworm can also affect the groin and thighs.

Treatment regimen

Use a few drops of allicin liquid added to your normal shampoo and use 2-3 times a week. At the same time take 2-4 capsules per day and this can be reduced down to 1 per day once you have gotten rid of the infection.

ROSACEA
Medical definition
This is a chronic inflammatory disease of the face in which the skin becomes abnormally flushed. It can become pustular and there may be associated keratinitis. Most common in women and the cause is now thought to be a type of parasite known as Demodex, which is found in the hair follicles and sebaceous glands. They resemble tiny worms and they are difficult to dislodge. It is also thought that the bacterium Helicobacter pylori *may be responsible for rosacea as well. Allicin will be able to destroy these parasites and bacterial infections.*

Treatment regimen
Apply 1 or 2 drops of allicin liquid or creme directly to the pustules once or twice per day. Also add 2 allicin powder capsules per day permanently to boost your immune system.

SARS (Severe acute respiratory syndrome)
ALL allicin formulations, powder, liquid and creme, have been requisitioned for testing by The National Institute for Health (NIH), the National Institute for Allergy and Infectious Diseases (NIAID) and The United States Army Military Research Institute for Infectious Diseases (USAMRIID). They are performing tests against a wide range of microbial species including SARS, West Nile virus, EEE (Eastern Equine Encephalitis), smallpox, Vaccinia and Variola species.

SCABIES
Medical definition
This is a skin infection caused by the mite sarcoptes scabiei. *Typified by severe itching especially at night. Characteristic red papules are caused by deposits of feces left by the mite which tunnels into the skin to start laying eggs. New hatched mites are easily spread to other people by direct contact. Intense itching represents an allergic reaction to the mite, its eggs and feces.*

The penis, nipples and the skin between the fingers are the most commonly affected areas. Normal treatment is with insecticides including Lindane and all sexual contacts and family members must be treated. Allicin has not been used to any great extent on treating scabies. As we have already seen, allicin can kill head lice so it would make sense to use the liquid in a soap to try and get rid of the mites. Currently, a soap formulation is only available in the UK and further work is underway to confirm its efficacy.

SHINGLES

This is another herpetic virus known as Herpes Zoster. A large dose of allicin capsules 6 to 10 per day should be taken for several moths to try and shift this resistant infection.

SINUSITIS
Medical definition

Sinusitis is an inflammation of the sinus cavities and may be caused by a variety of factors. Most recently Johns Hopkins Medical School has shown that recurrent sinusitis is often associated with a fungal infection. Other contributory factors will include food allergy reactions and inhalant allergy from existing medications.

Worldwide, millions of people suffer from sinus disease which causes symptoms like hay fever, runny nose, post nasal drip. People are encouraged to buy expensive OTC medications that may relieve symptoms for a short period but they soon relapse. Consequently, people are encouraged to have a minor operation to unplug the sinuses and remove all the infection built up. This is a relatively simple day surgery operation but it is rather uncomfortable! Unfortunately the symptoms usually recur after just a few months—since the fungal component of this infection keeps returning.

Allicin powder products have been used very successfully to get rid of this fungal element and if they are continued on a regular daily maintenance dose, the sinusitis stays away.

Treatment regimen

Take 1-3 capsules of Allisure allicin powder daily for 2 weeks followed by a maintenance dose of 1 capsule daily. You can also inhale the liquid formulation twice daily to add to the effect.

Testimonial

Mr. JH from Bexhill, UK, Mr. PD from Prescott, Arizona and Mrs. JAH from Oslo, Norway all had recurrent and persistent sinusitis. Having also had an operation to unblock the sinus cavities they still had the common symptoms including sneezing, runny nose and a constant feeling of being bunged up. They all tried using Allisure products and adopted the above protocol and gained excellent benefits.

SORE THROAT

A sore throat is caused by a variety of microbes including bacteria, virus and fungal species. As one of the most common infections known to man it is also one of the most troublesome, causing intense discomfort that can be only temporarily alleviated by local anaesthetics bought over the counter. However, we now have a simple and effective method of preventing a sore throat from causing discomfort and possibly leading onto a more serious infection—allicin capsules. All you need to do is take 2 or 3 capsules in one go and your sore throat will fade away and not get any worse. This is because allicin has this unique ability to kill both virus and bacteria at the same time.

TICK BORNE DISEASES

See parasites infestations

THRUSH

See Candida infections

TOOTHACHE

Toothache is almost always caused by an infection. An infection can be easily treated with allicin powder or liquid. In ancient times people used to cut up a clove of garlic and place it in or around the tooth abcess. Pain relief was usually immediate. This is what will happen if you either apply the liquid by rubbing a few drops in and around the painful area or alternatively, open up a capsule and rub a little allicin powder over the infected area.

TRAVELLERS' TUMMY

Remedies for travellers' tummy

The maxim that travel broadens the mind but loosens the bowels is all too true for up to half of us travelling to "high risk" areas, such as South America, Asia, Africa and parts of the Middle East (*Drugs and Therapeutics Bulletin, June 2002*). The familiar symptoms of "the runs" and cramps, accompanied by nausea and/or vomiting, can be both embarrassing and distressing. Consuming food or drink contaminated with bacteria, viruses, or parasites is usually to blame for travellers' diarrhea. Most cases are bacterial, with *E. coli* the prime suspect.

There are three approaches to coping with travellers' diarrhea: prevention (taking allicin powder capsules and probiotics before you go to ward off infection); self-treatment (taking a self-treatment kit with you this would also include a fluid replacement); and letting it run its course. The choice depends largely on your age, your general health, and the type of holiday envisaged. Most bouts of travellers' diarrhea clear up spontaneously in two to three days. But it's important to replace the fluid lost as dehydration can be dangerous, especially in the elderly and very young.

Aim for prevention if you have a condition that makes you prone to infection, for instance low immunity, diabetes, or an ailment that requires drugs to suppress stomach acid. In such cases it's probably worth discussing travel plans and the need for prophylactic antibiotics with your doctor. For most people, the US National Institutes of Health and the Centres for Disease Control advise against taking antibiotics for prevention of travellers' diarrhea.

The preventative approach is to take allicin powder capsules and a probiotic for a week before travelling. Trials have shown that probiotics can help restore the colonies of "friendly" bacteria that have been flushed out by infection and treatment and that allicin can both prevent bacterial infections and get rid of them quickly if you do pick one up.

"See a doctor if you have fever, blood and mucous in your stools, or diarrhea lasts more than five days."

If you choose the second option—self-treatment—there are several alternatives. Taking antibiotics after infection will usually shorten the duration of symptoms. Ciprofloxacin will deal with many of the culprit bugs but by adding allicin you get an extra benefit since the duration of the symptoms can be reduced to less than 6 hours. Resistance won't be a problem as the allicin can wipe out resistant cipro bugs. The allicin has the advantage of being able to work against viral or parasitic infections as well.

You should consult a doctor if there's any visible blood or mucous in your stool, or if the diarrhea persists for more than five days—diarrhea can be the signal for several serious conditions such as cholera, typhoid and parasitic infections.

Prevention

- Start taking allicin powder capsules and a probiotic 7 days before you travel
- Drink only "safe" drinks—clean water (boil water for 5 minutes, plus an extra minute for every 300 metres above sea level, or use bottled water) or commercial carbonated beverages
- Avoid ice cubes—they might be made from contaminated water
- Peel any fruit after washing in clean water
- Avoid salads and raw vegetables
- Eat only freshly cooked, hot food
- Steer clear of unpasteurised dairy products (e.g., milk, ice cream)
- Don't wade, paddle or swim in unfamiliar waters, as sewage outlets may discharge there and water-dwelling parasites can enter through the skin
- Don't go barefoot—some parasites enter through the feet
- Keep taking allicin powder capsules for 7 days after you return

TUBERCULOSIS

Medical definition

An infectious disease caused by the bacterium Mycobacterium tuberculosis. *Formerly known as consumption or wasting disease.*

Mycobacterium tuberculosis was identified in 1882 and exhibits a number of nodular lesions in the tissue. The disease can lay dormant for many years, but chronic infection is spread very easily by coughing or sneezing. Unfortunately, TB is once again on the increase as the number of cases reported in major international cities has more than doubled in the last 5 years. This is partly due to the influx of refugees and asylum seekers from parts of the world where TB is endemic, including countries like Mexico, Bosnia, Serbia, Russia, Afghanistan and several Middle Eastern countries.

It is reported that London is the TB capital of Europe and New York has set up special hospitals just to treat resistant cases. A broadcast on National Geographic TV Channel reports that in Russia they have 4 million people infected with TB, many of which are carrying drug-resistant strains who are just walking the streets spreading the pool of infection. Even worse, a large number of Russian prisoners are also infected and do not qualify for ANY treatment. So when they are released they can spread the disease further.

Recently, a number of strains of MDR TB were isolated from patients in a London teaching hospital. These re often treated by combinations of antibiotics including streptomycin and rifampicin. Any growth in the presence of an antimicrobial is significant with MDR *Mycobacterium tuberculosis* and growth was noted on all slopes where strains from these patients were treated with streptomycin. However, no growth was found on any of the slopes where strains were treated with allicin liquid.

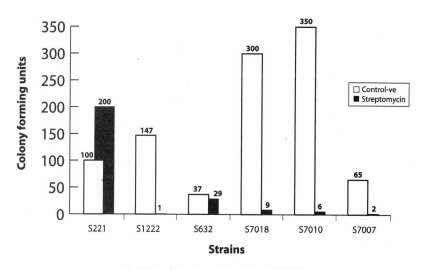

Activity of streptomycin against MDRTB

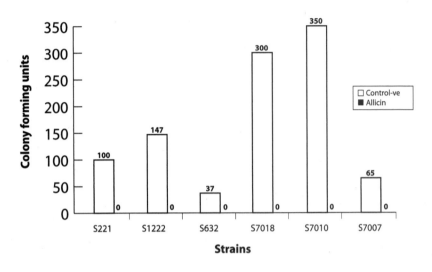

Activity of allicin against MDRTB
Graphs supplied by Dr. R. Cutler, UEL and Dr. P. Wilson, The Royal London Hospital

As illustrated above, all the strains isolated were completely killed off by allicin liquid. Since *Mycobacterium tuberculosis* tends to present mostly in the lungs we would expect allicin formulations to work very well. This is because allicin has a propensity for the lung tissue as it is very useful in chest infections and other diseases of the lung like asthma. Aside from this, allicin will boost the immune system substantially and allow your body to begin fighting off serious infections.

Treatment regimen

Begin by inhaling the allicin liquid several times a day. Dilute allicin liquid 1 part allicin to 2 parts water and take 10ml (two teaspoons full) every day. Add 6 capsules of allicin powder daily and continue this routine for a period of several weeks until any progress is noted.

VERRUCAE (Plantar warts)

Medical definition

Plantar warts (verrucae) occur on the soles of the feet and are often contracted in warm moist areas, particularly swimming pools and showers.

Treatment regimen and testimonial

While using allicin a couple of weeks ago, I noticed a verrucha on my heel. This is only the second I have ever had, the first was two years ago and lasted for months. I tried virtually every remedy on the market but to no avail (the little b's were multiplying!!), so I resorted to electrolysis treatment which, after several weekly visits to Sharon in Rye, worked. This time, I have used allicin liquid after washing once a day, and the offending article has already gone, and I might add, has not spread or caused any discomfort. Similarly, allicin did not kill the surrounding tissue.

Mrs. SB, Peasmarsh, East Sussex

VIRAL INFECTIONS

See the Common Cold

WARTS

Medical definition

A wart is a benign growth on the skin caused by infection with human papillomavirus. Common warts are firm horny papules, found mainly on the backs of the hands. Most will clear spontaneously within 2 years. Plane warts are flat and skin colored and therefore difficult to see; they are usually found on the face and may be present in very large numbers. Genital warts are frequently associated with other genital infections and affected women have an increased risk of developing cervical cancer.

Treatment regimen and testimonial

Mrs. DM from Sussex, England has used allicin creme to remove several warts from her head and hands. She has successfully used allicin creme applied once or twice daily by massaging a small amount into the surface of the wart. She says *"I found the creme easy to use and it has a pleasant smell. The successful treatment took me approximately 2 weeks and the warts had completely disappeared within 1 month."*

Miss SM from Florida was most upset to find a dozen or so little warts on the base of her foot. Her mom suggested that they use allicin liquid and applied a few drops to a bandage, which she placed over the warts. This was re-applied every day for no more than a week and to her delight and surprise the warts completely disappeared.

WOUNDS

Current research initiatives underway are showing that allicin formulations can help to heal wounds quickly and prevent infection. If an infection is present in a wound then allicin liquid, backed up by a normal dose of allicin powder capsules does appear to remove stubborn wound infections.

"This is unusual for me as I am a diabetic and find it very difficult to heal√I still have visible scars from when I was a teenager."

Personal Testimonial

I am a bit clumsy and have to admit that just about everytime I am out in the backyard I do something that causes me a minor injury! I get cuts on my fingers whilst trimming the hedges, I always get a splinter when moving wooden items around—sound familiar? Well, now I rountinely apply a little allicin liquid to the bandaid before I stick it over the wound.

A short while ago I got a nasty wooden splinter in my thumb. It immediately began to swell and was very painful. I managed to get the wood out but my thumb was beginning to balloon. So I just applied 2 drops of allicin liquid to the plaster and repeated this a few hours later. The pain had already gone and within a day the swelling was much better and I healed perfectly. This is also unusual for me as I am a diabetic and find it very difficult to heal—I still have visible scars from when I was a teenager. So this time my thumb healed perfectly. The old skin flaked away to reveal a perfectly healed wound with no scarring. I could have used a small dose of powder as an alternative but allicin liquid is really easy to use.

CHAPTER FOUR

How does allicin work and what else can it do?

Mechanism of action of allicin

This is a bit technical but well worth reading!

Inhibition of certain thiol-containing enzymes in the microorganisms by the rapid reaction of thiosulfinates with thiol groups was assumed to be the main mechanism involved in the antibiotic effect of allicin. Recently, we have studied the mechanism of action of pure allicin molecules with thiol groups in more detail. This study confirmed the ability of allicin to react with a model thiol compound (L-cysteine) to form the S-thiolation product S-allylmercaptocysteine. The identification of the thiolation product was proven by nuclear magnetic resonance as well as by mass spectroscopy.

The main antimicrobial effect of allicin is due to its interaction with important thiol-containing enzymes. In the amoeba parasite, allicin was found to strongly inhibit the cysteine proteinases, alcohol dehydrogenases, as well as the thioredoxin reductases enzymes which are critical for maintaining the correct redox state within the parasite. Inhibition of these enzymes was observed at rather low concentrations (<10 µg/mL). Allicin also irreversibly inhibited the well-known thiol-protease papain, the NADP$^+$-dependent alcohol dehydrogenase from *Thermoanaerobium brockii*, and the NAD$^+$-dependent alcohol dehydrogenase from horse liver. Interestingly, all three enzymes could be reactivated with thiol-containing compounds such as DTT, mercaptoethanol and glutathione.

Allicin also specifically inhibits other bacterial enzymes such as the acetyl-CoA-forming system, consisting of acetate kinase and phosphotransacetyl-CoA synthetase. The inhibition is noncovalent and reversible. (^{14}C) acetate incorporation into fatty acids of isolated plastids was inhibited by allicin with a 50% inhibitory concentration (I_{50} value) lower than 10 mM. Furthermore, allicin at bacteriostatic concentrations (0.2 to 0.5 mM) was found to partially inhibit, in *Salmonella typhimurium*, the DNA and protein synthesis, but the effect on RNA synthesis was immediate, suggesting that this could be a primary target of allicin action.

The condensation product of allicin, ajoene, which has a similar oxygenated sulfur group, has been shown to inhibit the proliferation of *Trypanosoma cruzi*, possibly by inhibition of phosphatidylcholine biosynthesis. Ajoene was also recently shown to inhibit phosphatidylcholine biosynthesis in the human pathogenic fungus *Paracoccidioides brasiliensis*. The inhibition capacities shown for ajoene clearly suggest that additional microbe-specific enzymes may also be targets for allicin.

At low concentrations, the inhibition of these enzymes may not be lethal, but sufficient to block the microbe's virulence. At slightly higher concentrations other enzymes, such as the dehydrogenases or thioredoxin reductases, may be affected and even a partial inhibition of these enzymes could be lethal for the microorganism.

All the above descriptions on the wide range of biological activities that allicin has, should have propelled this molecule into becoming a prime candidate for therapeutic use. Recently, it has been possible to patent the manufacture of allicin, produced in commercial quantities.

Having just listed an enormous range of medical benefits directly attributable to these real allicin formulations I have to admit that I could and probably will need to write several other books on the many and varied applications for this fantastic material.

The list of already proven herbal remedies that will gain extra impetus by the addition of allicin into their formulation is almost endless.

We already know that allicin can be safely added to the following list of "healthy raw materials" to make them even better:

- Vitamin C
- Probiotics
- Ginger
- Ellagic acid
- Echinacea
- Vitamins A and E
- Swedish flower pollen
- Black walnut hulls
- Wormwood
- Grapefruit seed extract
- Broccoli
- Garlic powder
- Digestive enzymes
- Hyaluronic acid
- Astralgus
- Ginkgo biloba
- Rosehips
- Gentian
- Hypericum
- Horse chestnut
- Ginseng
- Green tea
- Phosphatidyl serine

CHAPTER FIVE

Allicin and cancer prevention

It is estimated that one on three people will develop a type of cancer at some time in their life and cancer continues to account for around 25 percent of all deaths recorded each year. The causes are numerous and varied. Whilst only recognized as a separate disease in the last century, physicians have been diagnosing and treating "tumors" for thousands of years. Traditional Chinese medicine has always used garlic as a part of any treatment for the patients who suffered from a tumor or cancer. The search for compounds that prevent cancer has intensified with the mounting evidence that many types of cancer are caused or triggered by factors relating to lifestyle and environment. It is well-known and documented that allicin can strengthen the immune system, which is vitally important for fighting cancer. When I reviewed this important area of medicine, I was surprised and pleased to find a considerable amount of data already published that by taking allicin powder capsules regularly, you can receive some degree of protection against various stomach cancers and boost your CD4-T cell count. Interestingly, the medical community has known about this for years and is currently trying to establish which compounds are the most protective, since evidence also shows major benefits from diallyldisulphide, which is a common breakdown component of allicin powder. Many of the breakdown products from allicin have been tested for their inhibiting effect on cancer cells, and in most experiments inhibition of tumor growth was established.

Evidence from laboratory experiments and population surveys is presently inconclusive as to the preventative activity of allicin. Evidence also indicates that further research is warranted into the possible role of allicin in the prevention of cancer in humans.

Anticancer effects

In ancient times, garlic was used for the treatment of cancer of the uterus. Numerous reports, including several important epidemiological studies, have entered the scientific literature, asserting that garlic has a favorable effect on various forms of cancer. The following provides an overview of the current research and points of view concerning this very interesting special area of medicine.

Six decades ago, several statistical studies indicated that cancer occurs the least in those countries where garlic and onions are eaten regularly, such as France, Italy, the Netherlands, the Balkans, Egypt, India, and China. A review article published in 1936 referred to the connection between nutrition and cancer, and especially to the cancer growth-inhibiting effect of leek plants (Allium plants). The practising physicians of the time were very good observers, but almost nothing was known about the real background of this phenomenon. It was thought that the inhibitory action of garlic on putrefaction in the intestines, together with the secretion-stimulating effect, brought about detoxification and an increase in resistance. Stimulation of gastric juice secretion and restoration of the intestinal flora, combined with the resulting prevention of gastrointestinal autointoxication, may help to remove at least one of the possible causes of cancer. Garlic may therefore be useful as a cancer preventative agent, and its application as an anticancer "drug" is based on this assumption. More recently, this idea has again been pursued, not only in Europe, but also in the Third World countries, where the favorable effects of garlic for cancer are well known. For instance, the consumption of black or green tea, as well as of garlic, is known to be a culinary practice which inhibits tumorigenesis in the lung, forestomach, and esophagus. The only known study in which garlic has been used to treat patients with advanced stages of cancer was conducted by Spivak (1962). An aqueous garlic juice preparation was administered in doses of 0.2-2mL intravenously or 1-5mL intramuscularly daily for 3-7 days. Of 35 patients with cancer at various sites (lung, cervix, stomach, lower lip, mammary gland, larynx, and leukemia), 26 showed positive treatment results of differing degrees, though complete healing was not achieved in any case. There is a single-case report, however, of a man whose pituitary tumour shrank by 50% during the 5 months in which he ate 5-7 grams of fresh garlic daily. This was the first case ever reported of reduction of this type of tumor without chemotherapy or surgery.

Treatment regimen

Some notable success stories have been reported using allicin powder capsules, especially in Norway where patients with various types of cancer have dramatically improved their CD4-T cell count (remember this is a measure of how efficient your immune system is). Patients going through chemotherapy or radiotherapy tend to have very poorly functioning immune systems since they are effectively destroyed by treatment.

For 4 months, Mrs. EH from Norway had cell poisoning. Now her lymph cancer has gone, but she's continuing with allicin powder capsules and vitamins and minerals.

"When I got the cancer diagnosis, I became more interested in my diet. I thought it was very important to strengthen my immune system. Amongst other things, I found out that garlic is a significant antioxidant which prevents the body from deteriorating," says Elsa.

Since it is difficult to ingest large amounts of fresh garlic, Elsa chose to invest in capsules. She started with two per day, but later increased this to six per day. She reports, *"Then I was in control (in the summer).*

My blood count was very good. Personally, I think it was due to the allicin." There are many garlic products on the market, but Elsa chose to take one that can gurantee real allicin.

Elsa has now been without cell poisoning for over a year. She regularly goes to the doctor for check-ups but gets happier because her blood count gets better every time. She praises the doctor and the hospital because she got such good service.

Elsa believes that a healthy lifestyle without smoking and alcohol, together with Weissin, vitamins and mineral supplements has given her a good immune system. Of course, she is concerned that the cancer may come back, but she chooses to think positively. She thanks God that she is well.

Anticancer Effects: Active Compounds

From the many publications that have been reviewed, it is apparent that the anticancer effects of garlic are likely due to allicin and allicin-derived compounds as well as unidentified compounds not related to allicin. The following is a summary of the evidence for possible active compounds.

1) Epidemiological studies from six different countries have consistently shown that garlic consumption is associated with decreased risk of gastrointestinal cancer. Since garlic is mainly eaten cooked (allinase inactivated) in most of these countries, allicin may not be necessary to achieve significant cancer reduction.

2) A major decrease in incidence of gastric cancer in China, particularly where large amounts of allicin-yielding fresh garlic are eaten, is associated with the antibiotic effects of garlic and its thiosulfinates (allicin) toward decreasing the amount of nitrate-reducing bacteria in the stomach, hence the amounts of carcinogenic nitrosamines formed. Therefore, allicin does appear to have an important role in prevention of gastric cancer.

3) Animal studies have indicated the importance of allicin, since dietary fresh garlic (but not allinase-inhibited garlic), greatly decreased breast cancer incidence in mice.

A large number of animal studies with allicin-derived diallyl disulfide and diallyl sulfide, most using very large doses (100-200mg/kg), have shown positive effects toward decreasing carcinogen-induced cancer. Although allicin itself has not been tested, these studies indicate that allicin-derived compounds have the ability to affect cancer incidence.

The new allicin containing products also naturally form all the beneficial components that are not stabilized when fresh or cooked garlic is used.

CHAPTER SIX

Conclusion

In the last three decades we have seen several viral and bacterial epidemics which took place at a time where we would have expected the eradication of many infectious diseases. There are many hypotheses to explain this paradox:

- Is it the hygiene theory—extensive use of wide-spread and excessively potent antibiotics which eliminate protective infecting agents?
- Is it the widespread use of vaccines?
- Is it a mistake or a terrorist act of leakage of viral mutant from research or other laboratories?

Regardless of the cause, globalization and long-distance flights make it easy to spread disease to the far reaches of the globe.

In the twenty-first century, we have already identified a number of infectious organisms that can and will present a major problem to patients, physicians, healthcare workers and administrators all over the world. These will include:

MRSA (sensitive to allicin)

MDR Tuberculosis (sensitive to allicin)

VRE Vancomycin resistant enterococcus (sensitive to allicin)

PRSP Penicillin resistant Strep. pneum. (not yet tested)

VRSA Vancomycin resistant Staphylococcus aureus (sensitive to allicin)

VISA & GISA (Glycopeptide intermediate resistant *Staphylococcus aureus*—1st case in UK in Dec 2002 sensitive to allicin)

With MRSA now reported in the "healthy community," the writing is already on the wall. We need something that can take on these superbugs and win the battle for us. We need to reduce our dependence on pharmaceutical antibiotics, or at least make them more effective. If we don't, these powerful microbes will take over.

Already, infectious disease is a bigger killer than heart disease or cancer. The devastating effect of infectious organisms is disease and suffering through disability, disfigurement and premature death. The above organisms cannot be easily treated by anything the all-powerful pharmaceutical industry has to offer. Shockingly, effective even before they hit the market, the latest antibiotics are unable to kill certain species of bacteria.

"Allicin is Nature's antibiotic, antifungal and antiviral. It could change the course of history!"

We have seen the international panic over SARS, and now MRSA is spreading through the healthy population. This is frightening, but doctors routinely find organisms like *E. coli, Helicobacter pylori, Tuberculosis, Herpes, Acinetobacter, Cryptosporidium, Camplylobacter, HIV, Salmonella, Cholera*, flesh-eating bacteria and others that are becoming multi-drug resistant. Consequently, thousands of people die needlessly when treatment is simple.

Allicin is nature's antibiotic, antifungal and antiviral. It could change the course of history! But we must all pull together to ensure that people can obtain it—in whatever form they need. Allicin has the capability to save many lives—perhaps even yours!

Here is my guarantee. Even if you are a relatively fit and healthy individual with no other complicating diseases, YOU will notice a difference when you start taking allicin powder capsules. Within 3 weeks, you will feel different, you will be detoxing your system and you will notice the change in your general health and well-being. You will be buying into protection and prevention, and any doctor will tell you prevention is always better than treatment. So go try some real allicin today. Your body needs it!

Bibliography

Oxford Medical Dictionary Fourth Edition

Darbyshire B., Henry R.J., *Differences in fructan content and synthesis in some Allium species, New Phytol. 87 (1981) 249-256.*

Koch H.P., Lawson L.D., *Garlic, the science and therapeutic application of Allium sativum L. and related species*, in: Retford D.C. (Ed.), Williams and Wilkins, Baltimore, 1996, pp. 1-233.

Cavallito C., Bailey J.H., *Allicin, the antibacterial principle of Allium sativum. Isolation, physical properties and antibacterial action*, J. Am. Chem. Soc. 66 (1944) 1944-1952.

Block E., *The chemistry of Garlic and Onion*, Sc. Am. 252 (1985) 94-99.

Stoll A., Seebeck E., *Chemical investigations of alliin, and the specific principle of garlic*, Adv. Enzymol. 11 (1951) 377-400.

Ellmore G.S., Feldberg R.S., *Alliin lyase localization in bundle sheaths of garlic clove (Allium sativum)*, Am. J. Bat. 81(1994) 89-94.

Rabinkov A., Xiao-Zhu Z., Grafl G., Galili G., Mirelman D., *Alum lyase (alliinase) from garlic (Allium sativum):Biochemical characterization and cDNAcloning*, Appl.Biochem.Biotechnol. 48 (1994) 149-171.

Van Damme 5.3.24., Smeets K., Torrekens S., Van Leaven F., Peumans W.J., *Isolation and characterization of alliinase cDNA clones from garlic (Alliumsativum L.) and related species*, Eur.J. Biochem. 209 (1992) 751-757.

Rabinkov A., Wilchek M., Mirelman D., *Alumnae (alum lyase) from garlic (Allium sativum) is glycosylated at ASN146 and forms a complex with a garlic mannosespecific lectin*, Glyco conj. 3. 12 (1995) 690-698.

Uchida Y., Takahashi T., Sato N., *The characteristics of the antibacterial activity of garlic*, Jpn J. Antibiotics 28 (1975) 638-642.

Celiini L, Di Campli B., Masulli M., Di Bartolomeo S., Aliocati N., *Inhibition of Helicobacter pylori by garlic extract (Allium sativum)*, FEMS Immenol. Med. Micrbiol 13 (1996) 273-277.

Gonzalez-Fandos F., Garcia-Lopez Mi.., Sierra Mi., Otero A., *Staphylococcal growth and enterotoxins (A-D) and thermonuclease synthesis in the presence of dehydrated garlic*, J. Appl. Bacteriol. 77 (1994) 549-552.

Girnenez MA., Solanes RE., Girneriez D.F., *Growth of Clostridium botulinum in media with garlic*, Rev. Argent. Microbioi. 20 (1988) 17-24.

Holzgartner H, Schmidt U, Kuhn U Congress Abstract Eur Jnl Clin Res 3A 1992:8.

Brosche T and Platt D (1991) *Garlic BMJ*; 303; 785.

Rabinkov A.,. Miron T., Konsrantinovski L., Wilchek M., Mirelman D., Weiner L., *The mode of action of allicin: trapping of radicals and interaction with thiol containing proteins*, Biochim. Biophys. Acts 1379 (1998) 233-244.

Abdullah TH, Kirkpatrick DH, Carter J; *Enhancement of Natural Killer Cell activity in AIDS patients*; D Z Onkologie 21;52-53.

Josling P, *Advances in Natural Therapy* (2001) 18; 189-193.

Steinmetz *et al.*, (1994), *Vegetable fruit and colon cancer in The IOWA Women's Health Study*. Am. J. Epidemiol. 139: 1-15.

Eccles R., *Common Cold Centre* Cardiff.

Koch and Lawson in *Garlic—The Science and Therapeutic Application of Allium Sativum L and Related Species*. Williams & Wilkins; 1996.

Ankri & Mirelman. *Microbes Infect.* 1999; 2:125-129.

Hanley & Fenwick. *J Plant Foods*. 1985; 6:211-238.

Data on file. Garlic Centre, East Sussex, UK.

Appendix

Table 1

Fungal and dermatophyte infections against which Allisure® allicin powder, creme or liquid may be effective

* Athlete's foot	* Geotrichum candidum	* Kloeckera apiculata
* Candida albicans	* Trichoderma hamatum	* Oospora lactis
* Aspergillus fumigatus	* Trichophyton cerebriforme	* Penicillium notatum
* Aspergillus niger	* Trichophyton granulosum	* Cryptococcus neoformans
* Rhizopus nigricans	* Trichophyton terrestre	* Microsporum canis
* Mucor racemosus	* Malbranchea pulchella	* Epidermaphyton mentagrophytes
* Didium lactus	* Chrysosporium tropicum	* Aspergillus flavus
* Coccidioides immitis (Valley Fever)	* Microsporum canis	* Parracoccoides brasiliensis
* Torilopsum spp.	* Aspergillus parasiticus	* Ringworm
* Rhodotorula spp.	* Aspergillus ochraceus	* Histoplasma capsulatum
* Trichosporon spp.	* Penicillum spp.	
* Auxarthron zufiianum	* Microsporum gypseum	* Direct observation reported in scientific literature or personal communication to the author
* Uncinocarpus resii	* Saccharomyces spp.	
* Fusarium laceratum		

Table 2

Bacterial infections against which Allisure® allicin powder, creme or liquid may be effective (all with very low concentrations required to prevent infection).

This very wide range of sensitive bacterial species shows just how allicin can help to revolutionize the treatment of infectious diseases.

* Acinetobacter baumii	* Mycobacterium leprae	* Helicobacter pylori
* Acinetobacter calcoaceticus	* Mycobacterium bovis	* Streptococcus pyogenes (flesh eating bacteria)
* Escherichia coli	* Mycobacterium kansasii	
* Bacillus cereus	* Helicobacter pylori	* Klebsiella aerogenes
* Bacillus subtilis	* Cornyebacterium spp.	* Saccharomyces cerevisiae
* Campylobacter jejuni	* Pasteurella spp.	* Meningitis
* Camplylobacter fetus	* Cryptococcus spp.	* Cholera
* Camplylobacter coli	* Salmonella typhimurium	* Listeria monocytogenes
* Campylobacter doylei		
* Campylobacter hyointestinalis	* Salmonella dublinii	* Enterococcus faecium
* Campylobacter ureolyticus	* Salmonella enteriditis	* Pseudomonas aeroginosa
	* Shigella	
* Campylobacter mucosalis	* Bacillus anthracis	* Proteus mirabilis
* Campylobacter helveticus	* MRSA (Methicillin resistant staphylococcus aureus)	* Nesseria Gonorrhea
		* Chlostridium perfringens
* Citrobacter spp.	* GISA (Glycopeptide intermediate resistant staphylococcus aureus)	* Chlamydia
* Hafnia spp		* Hemophilus Influenza
* Provindencia spp.	* VISA (Vancomycin intermediate resistant staphylococcus aureus)	* Direct observation reported in scientific literature or personal communication to the author
* Micrococcus		
* Mycobacterium tuberculosis	* Staphylococcus aureus in skin disease	

Table 3

Viral infections against which Allisure® allicin powder, liquid and creme may be effective.

* Influenza A	* Cytomegalovirus	Croup
* Common Rhinovirus (Cold infection)	* Pox virus	Chicken Pox
	* Parvovirus	* Vaccinia virus
* Influenza B	* Herpes Simplex Type 1 & 2 (Cold Sores)	* Variola virus
* Coxiella burnetii (Q-Fever)		* Vesicular Stomatitis virus
	* Herpes Zoster (Shingles)	
* Pneumonia		* Direct observation reported in scientific literature or personal communication to the author
Severe acute Respiratory Syndrome (SARS)	Warts	
	Flu	

Table 4

Parasitic disease against which Allisure® allicin powder, liquid or creme may be useful.

* Amebic dysentery	* Tapeworms	Lung flukes
* Cryptosporidium	* Echinococcus	* Head lice
* Giardiasis	* Trichomonas	* Lyme Disease
Toxoplasmosis	* Round worm (Ascaris strongyloides)	* Direct observation reported in scientific literature or personal communication to the author
* Leishmaniasis	* Shistomiasis	
* Malaria	* Filariasis	
* Oxyuriasis (pin worm infestation)	Intestinal flukes	
* Hookworm	Liver flukes	

Table 5

Other diseases against which Allisure® allicin powder, liquid or creme may be useful.

* Takayasu's disease	* Multiple Sclerosis	* Pneumonia
* Elevated blood pressure	Chronic fatigue syndrome	* Genital herpes
* Elevated cholesterol	Fibromyalagia	* Direct observation reported in scientific literature or personal communication to the author
Raynaud's disease	* Labyrinthritis	
* Rocky Mountain Spotted Fever	* Giardiasis	

INDEX

A

Acinetobacter   12, 150

Acne   32, 42

AIDS   33, 73, 98, 120

Alcohol   55, 61, 129, 141, 147

Allergic reaction   84, 123, 131

Animal bites   36

Antibiotics   7-8, 22, 41, 45-46, 50, 55, 57, 79, 100, 112-113, 115, 117, 121, 124, 134, 136, 150

Antioxidants   77, 98,

Arthritis   37, 77, 126

Aspergillus   51, 154

Asthma   38, 8, 97, 137

Athlete's foot   38, 39

B

Bacillus subtilis   155

Bacterial infection   8, 27, 40, 44, 46, 99, 112, 129, 134

Bad breath   45

Bites   36, 105, 109, 113

Bladder infection   47

Boils   50, 113

C

Campylobacter   155

Cancer   12, 77-78, 95-96, 98, 122, 138, 145-148

Candida albicans   32, 39, 52-55, 76, 82, 121, 154

Canker sores   56

Chlamydia   155

Clostridium   155

Clove   16, 19, 120, 133,

Colds   15, 63, 72, 75, 97

Cold sores   62

Cortisone   62, 87

Croup   156

Cryptosporidium   73, 120

Cuts   75, 139

D

Dandruff   73

Demodex   130

Dengue fever   80

Dermatophytes   82

Diabetes   49, 74, 133

Diaper rash   76

Diarrhea   76

Drugs   38, 47, 81, 128

Dysentery   7

E

E. Coli   46

Ear infections   78

Ebola   80

Echinacea   143

Eczema   42, 81

F

Flesh eating bacteria	150, 155
Flu	63
Fungal infection	6, 11, 31, 38, 46, 74, 76, 78, 121, 129, 131

G

Garlic	6, 11
Gastritis	123
Genital herpes	62
Giardia lamblia	120
Gingivitis (Gum disease)	83

H

Head lice	90, 102, 131
Helicobacter pylori	11, 41, 43, 89, 95, 122, 123
Hemorrhagic fever	80
Hepatitis	7, 94-95, 70
Herpes	62, 95, 109
High blood pressure	36, 47

I

Immune system	28
Impetigo	99
Influenza	65
Insecticides	90-91, 95, 131
Irritable bowel syndrome	37, 100
Itchy skin	81

J– K

Klebsiella	41
Kidneys	46

L

Lactobacillus	101
Lindane	131
Lung infection	63
Lyme	157

M

Malaria	15, 105, 107, 128
Mercury	31, 94
Microbes	7, 36, 132, 150
Mites	106, 130
Mosquitoes	11, 15, 105
MRSA	12, 42, 110-119, 150
Mycobacterium	41, 135, 137

N

Nail fungus	83
Nausea	133

O – P

Parasites	11, 31, 40, 73, 103, 105, 119-120
Penicillin	114
Peptic ulcer	121, 123
Pneumonia	11, 34, 63, 114
Plaque	8, 82-83, 126-127
Proteus	41, 43
Pseudomonas	43
Psoriasis	126-129

Q – R

Rash	67, 76
Respiratory disease	86
Rhinitis	45
Ringworm	39, 129
Rocky Mountain Spotted Fever	12
Rosacea	130

S

Salmonella	41, 43, 101, 142, 150
Scabies	130
Shigella	7, 41
Shingles	131
Sinus	45, 56, 64, 131
Sore throat	38, 63, 71, 89, 132
Staphylococcus	10, 32, 41, 43, 64, 81, 110
Stomach acid	20, 121, 133
Streptococcus	32, 43-44, 56, 64

T

Thrush	50-56, 132
Trichophyton	39, 129
Tuberculosis	7, 15, 22, 41, 43, 135, 149, 150
Typhus	7, 22

U – V

Ulceration	103
Vaginal infection	51
Viruses	8, 31, 63, 65, 80, 94, 122, 133
Vitamin C	55, 143

W – Z

Warts	138-139
Wounds	30, 46, 116, 139
Yeast infection	50, 52, 83

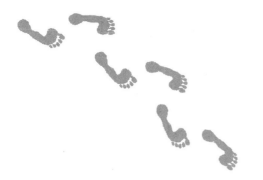

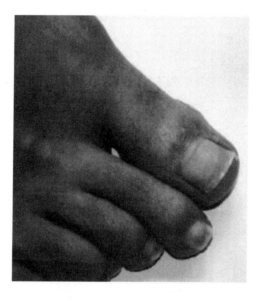

Success with that fungal nail infection using allicin creme (or liquid) has completely healed the big toe. This took just 6 weeks applying a small dab of creme each day.